Other Examination Preparation Books Published by Petroc Press:

Balcombe	*Notes for the MRCP Part I*	190060342X
Bateson	*Basic Tests in Gastroenterology*	1900603772
Bateson	*MCQs in Clinical Gastroenterology*	1900603519
Bateson	*MCQs on the Upper Digestive Tract*	1900603373
Bateson & Stephen	*MCQs in Gastroenterology*	1900603403
Black & Kelleher	*MCQs in Anaesthesiology*	1900603454
Chakravorty	*Visual Aids to the MRCP Examination*	0792388739
Chong & Wong	*Survival Kit for MRCP Part II*	1900603063
Edgell	*Preparing for MRCP Part II Cardiology*	0792388690
Green	*More MCQs for Finals*	079238928X
Green (Ed.)	*The MRCPsych Study Manual: 2nd edn*	1900603527
Helmy & Mokbel	*Preparing for the PLAB Part 1*	1900603721
Hogston	*MCQs for the MRCoG Part II*	1900603551
Kubba *et al.*	*MCQs for MFFP Part I*	1900603004
Levi	*Basic Notes in Psychiatry: 2nd edn*	1900603306
Levi	*Basic Notes in Psychotherapy*	1900603500
Levi	*Basic Notes in Psychopharmacology: 2nd edn*	1900603608
Levi	*MCQs in Psychiatry for MRCPsych*	1900603853
Levi	*PMPs for the MRCPsych Part II*	079238993X
Levi	*SAQs for the MRCPsych*	0746200994
Levy & Riordan Eva	*MCQs in Optics and Refraction*	1900603225
Levy & Riordan Eva	*MCQs for the FRCOphth*	1900603276
Levy & Riordan Eva	*MCQs for the MRCOphth*	1900603179
Mokbel	*MCQs in Applied Basic Medical Sciences*	1900603756
Mokbel	*MCQs in General Surgery*	1900603101
Mokbel	*MCQs in Neurology*	0792388577
Mokbel *et al.*	*MCQs for the MRCP Part I*	1900603071
Mokbel	*Operative Surgery and Surgical Topics for the FRCS/MRCS*	1900603705
Mokbel	*SAQs in Clinical Surgery-in-General for the FRCS*	190060390X
Ross & Emmanuel	*MCQs on Antimicrobial Therapy*	1900603411
Ross & Emmanuel	*MCQs in Medical Microbiology for MRCP*	0792388836
Ross & Emmanuel	*MCQs in Medical Microbiology and Infectious Diseases*	1900603365
Ross & Emmanuel	*MCQs in Microbiology and Infection for FRCS*	1900603152
Rymer & Higham	*Preparing for the DRCoG*	1900603012
Sandler & Sandler	*MCQs in Cardiology for MRCP Pt I*	0792389999
Sandler & Sandler	*MCQs in Cardiology*	0792389387
Sandler & Sandler	*More MCQs in Cardiology for MRCP Pt I*	0792388402
Sikdar	*MCQs in Basic Sciences for MRCPsych Pt II*	190060356X

Obtainable from all good booksellers or, in case of difficulty, from Plymbridge Distributors Limited, Plymbridge House, Estover Road, PLYMOUTH, Devon PL6 7PZ

Tel.   01752–202300
FAX   01752–202333

MCQs for the MRCS

K. M. Mokbel MB, BS(London), FRCS(Eng), FRCS(Gen)

Senior Registrar
Department of Surgery
The Royal Hospital of St. Bartholomew,
The Royal London Hospital and
The London Chest Hospital NHS Trust
London

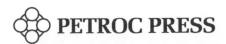

PETROC PRESS

Petroc Press, an imprint of LibraPharm Limited

Distributors

Plymbridge Distributors Limited, Plymbridge House, Estover Road, Plymouth PL6 7PZ, UK

First edition 2000

Published in the United Kingdom by
LibraPharm Limited
Gemini House
162 Craven Road
NEWBURY
Berks
RG14 5NR

A catalogue record for this book is available from the British Library

ISBN 1 900603 82 9

Printed and bound in the United Kingdom by
MPG Books Ltd, Bodmin, Cornwall

Contents

Introduction

The MRCS examination aims to test a broad range of knowledge in basic and clinical sciences at an early stage of training in surgery. The format of the examination is influenced by the large number of candidates and the necessity to provide a uniform and standard method of assessment.

The multiple-choice question (MCQ) format, as part of this examination, has come to stay. It provides a standardised method of assessment covering a broad spectrum of knowledge. It also exposes both areas of weakness, as well as areas of strength, in the candidates' knowledge, and thus provides a fine stone to sharpen the knife of his or her knowledge.

The written part of the MRCS examination consists of two MCQ papers. The first paper covers, primarily, core modules including anatomy, physiology, clinical chemistry, pathology, microbiology, oncology, trauma and principles of surgery. The second paper covers systemic modules including gastrointestinal, vascular, cardiothoracic, paediatric, breast, endocrine, urological, orthopaedic and plastic subspecialities. However, there is a significant degree of overlap between the two papers and the second paper almost always contains questions covering basic sciences such as anatomy and pathology. Each MCQ paper contains approximately 45 multiple true/false questions and 10 extended matching questions (EMQs).

This book contains more than 350 questions with answers and explanations arranged in four mock examination practice papers (two core module and two system module papers). The examination is positively marked (no mark is deducted for an incorrect answer) and a score of 75% or more is regarded as being satisfactory. Many of the questions included in this book have appeared in previous examination papers (memory-retrieved) in order to familiarise candidates with the standard and nature of the MRCS examination.

I hope that this book will be both stimulating and helpful to candidates preparing for the examination.

London, 2000   K. M.

Core Modules Paper A

Questions

Q1 In a 60-year-old man with the syndrome of inappro-priate ADH secretion the following results are strongly consistent with the diagnosis:

A. Serum sodium 115 mmol/litre
B. Urine osmolality 600 mmol/kg
C. Serum osmolality 300 mmol/kg
D. A biochemical response to fluid restriction
E. Urine sodium 15 mmol/litre

Q2 The serum potassium of a 60-year-old woman was found to be 2.2 mmol/litre. The following conditions may explain this abnormal result:

A. Frusemide therapy
B. Addison's disease (not associated with hypovolaemic shock)
C. Villous adenoma of the rectum
D. Diarrhoea
E. Untreated diabetic keto-acidosis
F. Metabolic alkalosis
G. Succinyl choline administration

Q3 The thyrocervical trunk usually:

A. Arises from the second part of the subclavian artery
B. Lies directly anterior to the stellate ganglion
C. Gives off the suprascapular artery
D. Gives off the deep cervical artery
E. Gives off the superior intercostal artery

Q4 When exploring the wrist the following structures are found to lie superficial to the flexor retinaculum:

A. The ulnar nerve
B. The ulnar artery
C. The median nerve
D. The palmar cutaneous branch of the ulnar nerve
E. Flexor digitorum superficialis

Q5   When performing a pneumonectomy from the posterior approach:

A. The phrenic nerve passes anterior to the lung root
B. The vagus nerve passes anterior to the lung root
C. The oesophagus lies behind the left atrium
D. The azygous vein arches over the right main bronchus
E. The hemizygous vein arches over the right main bronchus

Q6   The following statements refer to the inguinal canal:

A. The posterior wall is formed by transversus abdominis
B. The canal allows the passage of the round ligament of the uterus to the labium majus
C. It transmits the ilio-hypogastric nerve
D. The superficial ring lies directly anterior to the deep ring in the newborn
E. On coughing, the canal becomes almost closed

Q7   Considering cell response to injury:

A. In hypoxic cells K^+ is retained in the cells and Na^+ escapes from them
B. Hypoxia does not lead to the formation of powerful oxidants in cells due to lack of oxygen
C. In hydropic degeneration the cells are typically dehydrated
D. Fatty change is a recognised cell response to damage by poisons or hypoxia
E. A free radical is a molecule that contains an odd number of electrons

Q8   In the base of the skull:

A. Foramen spinosum transmits the facial nerve
B. Foramen magnum transmits the vertebral arteries
C. Foramen rotundum transmits the greater petrosal nerve
D. Foramen ovale transmits the maxillary nerve
E. Stylomastoid foramen transmits the glossopharyngeal nerve

Q9   In wound healing:

A. When collagen is synthesised hydroxyproline and hydroxylysine are incorporated directly into the collagen molecule
B. Collagen lysis is increased in infected wounds
C. The wound weakens in scurvy due to increased activity of collagenase
D. When using absorbable sutures, the wound strength progressively increases to maximum from the time of suturing
E. The inflammatory response to suture insertion is greater for monofilamentous nylon than for catgut

Q10   Oncogenes:

A. Are genes capable of causing cancer
B. Have been isolated from about 75% of human cancers
C. Products are protein kinases in about 50% of viral oncogenes
D. May uncouple the intranuclear mechanisms involved in growth control from the need for an external stimulus
E. Include growth suppressor genes

Q11   Unfractionated heparin:

A. May cause thrombocytopenia
B. Anticoagulation is best monitored by measuring INR
C. Is antagonised by protamine sulphate
D. Has longer duration of action than low-molecular-weight heparin
E. Is usually given as 5000 units subcutaneously twice daily to treat an established DVT

Q12   Warfarin:

A. Anticoagulation is effective 24 hours after the first dose
B. Is well absorbed from the alimentary tract
C. Has a half-life of about 6 hours
D. Action is terminated mainly by renal excretion
E. Metabolism by the liver is induced by cimetidine

Q13   Familial hypocalcuric hypercalcaemia:

A. Is inherited in an autosomal recessive fashion
B. Is characterised by increased urinary excretion of calcium
C. Is a recognised cause of acute pancreatitis
D. Is characterised by elevated serum parathyroid hormone (PTH)
E. May present at any age
F. Can be excluded if both parents are unaffected on blood sampling

Q14   Stored cross-matched blood:

A. pH gradually rises
B. Potassium concentration gradually increases
C. Rapidly loses clotting factors
D. May cause hypothermia when transfused
E. Commonly causes hypercalcaemia after transfusion

Q15   The complications of massive blood transfusion include:

A. Air embolism
B. Hyperkalaemia
C. Thrombocythaemia
D. Disseminated intravascular coagulopathy (DIC)
E. Metabolic alkalosis

Q16   In a normal mammalian cell:

A. There is 21 pairs of somatic chromosomes and two pairs of sex
   chromosomes
B. Meiosis produces four haploid cells from one diploid cell
C. Chromosomes are most easily visible by light microscopy during
   the interphase
D. The nucleus has a double membrane
E. Gametes are diploid
F. DNA replication occurs during the S-phase of cell cycle

Q17   Causes of thrombocytopenia include:

A. Heparin therapy
B. Haemolytic uraemic syndrome
C. Disseminated intravascular coagulopathy
D. Splenectomy (assuming no significant blood loss)
E. Sarcoidosis

Q18   In haemophilia A:

A. Prothrombin time is prolonged
B. A factor VIII C level of 20% is adequate for major surgery
C. Desmopressin can elevate factor VIII levels three-fold
D. The half-life of injected factor VIII is 24 hours
E. The inheritance is X-lined recessive

Q19   Recognised consequences of endotoxic shock include:

A. Adult respiratory distress syndrome (ARDS)
B. Gastrointestinal haemorrhage
C. Hypothermia
D. Interstitial oedema
E. Hypertrophic obstructive cardiomyopathy

Q20   The following are synthetic absorbable sutures:

A. Polyester   (Dacron)
B. Polyamide   (Nylon)
C. Polydioxanone   (PDS)
D. Polypropylene   (Prolene)
E. Polyglycolic acid (Dexon)

Q21   In local anaesthesia, lignocaine:

A. Causes a rapid inflow of Na^+ into excitable cells
B. Is more effective if injected into an inflamed area
C. Maximal safe dose is 10 mg per kg
D. Is shorter acting than buvicaine
E. Can cause a cardiac arrest

Q22   Pulse oximetry:

A. Usually uses six wavelengths of light
B. Is based on Beer's law
C. Using an ear probe, is more precise than using a finger probe
D. Mean error is less than 5%
E. Readings are not influenced by nail polish when using finger probes

Q23   Autoclaving:

A. Utilises moist steam at 100°C and a pressure of $5\,lb/in^2$
B. Is the most frequently used method of sterilisation of surgical instruments
C. Requires 3 hours for sterilisation
D. Is primarily used to sterilise glassware
E. Does not kill clostridial spores

Q24   Diathermy:

A. Means 'heating through'
B. Current follows the pathway of minimal resistance
C. Causes less surrounding tissue damage when used in the monopolar form
D. Plate should be placed as far as possible from the operating field
E. Is a recognised cause of explosions in the operating room

Q25   Mammography:

A. Has a 98% sensitivity
B. Is valuable in assessing breast lumps in women under the age of 35 years
C. As a screening tool, has reduced breast cancer mortality in women over the age of 50 years
D. Usually shows round macrocalcifications in patients with DCIS
E. Does not significantly increase the risk of breast cancer if performed annually

Q26   With reference to the lymphatic spread of breast cancer:

A. The sentinel node is the first node to receive lymph from the area containing the primary tumour
B. Level III axillary nodes are located behind the pectoralis minor muscle
C. Level I axillary nodes are located behind the pectoralis minor muscle
D. Lateral breast tumours are more likely to metastasise to the axillary nodes than medial tumours
E. The axillary node status is the best single prognostic indicator

Q27 The following have been shown to reduce breast cancer mortality:

A. Screening mammography in women over the age of 50 years
B. Axillary clearance in women with early breast cancer
C. Adjuvant tamoxifen therapy in pre-menopausal women with invasive breast cancer
D. Adjuvant cytotoxic chemotherapy in node positive pre-menopausal patients
E. Post-operative radiotherapy in post-menopausal patients with early invasive breast cancer

Q28 Anterior shoulder dislocation:

A. Is less common than posterior shoulder dislocation
B. Is usually subcoracoid
C. Usually presents with the arm in the adduction position
D. Is a recognised cause of axillary nerve palsy
E. Can be treated using Kocher's manoeuvre

Q29 Carpal tunnel syndrome:

A. Is a recognised complication of rheumatoid arthritis (RA)
B. Is frequently caused by a cervical rib
C. Spares the abductor pollicis brevis
D. Diagnosis is confidently made with the use of electrophysiological tests
E. Is treated by division of the extensor retinaculum

Q30 Cutaneous melanoma:

A. Is often associated with p53
B. Arises in a pre-existing mole in 40% of cases
C. Prognosis is independent of Breslow's thickness
D. Is radiosensitive
E. Prognosis is independent of sex

Q31   The oxygen dissociation curve is shifted to the right in:

A. Polycythaemia rubra vera
B. Chronic anaemia
C. Pyrexia
D. Respiratory alkalosis
E. States of decreased concentration of 2,3-diphosphogylcerate (2,3-DPG) inside the red cell

Q32   In metabolic acidosis:

A. There is a negative base excess
B. HCO_3^- is the main intracellular buffer
C. Proteins and phosphates are the main extracellular buffer
D. Compensation occurs by an increase in alveolar ventilation
E. Bicarbonate infusion is the mainstay of treatment

Q33   Recognised causes of hypokalaemia include:

A. Villous adenoma of the rectum
B. Captopril therapy
C. Conn's syndrome
D. Spironolactone therapy
E. Diabetes insipidus

Q34   Iron:

A. Is absorbed primarily in the stomach
B. Binds to apoferritin in enterocytes
C. In the ferric form (Fe^{3+}) is more easily absorbed than in the ferrous form (Fe^{2+})
D. Absorption is impaired by vitamin C
E. Body stores are best represented by serum transferrin levels

Q35   Cardiac tamponade in trauma patients:

A. Causes a rise in JVP
B. Is characterised by loud heart sounds
C. Is effectively treated by pericardiocentesis in most cases
D. Is a recognised indication for thoracotomy
E. Can be accurately diagnosed with two-dimensional echocardiography
F. Causes Kussmaul's sign
G. Is a recognised cause of pulsus paradoxus > 10 mm Hg

Q36   In trauma patients, the indications for immediate thoracotomy in the accident and emergency department include:

A. Initial chest drain insertion yields 800 ml of blood
B. Flail chest with cardiopulmonary arrest
C. Massive abdominal haemorrhage
D. Pneumomediastinum
E. Penetrating injury causing cardiac tamponade and EMD

Q37   Post-operative pulmonary atelectasis:

A. Incidence is decreased by pre-operative breathing exercises
B. Is mainly treated by antimicrobials
C. Is a common cause of post operative pyrexia
D. May be treated by flexible bronchoscopy
E. Incidence is increased by epidural analgesia in patients undergoing laparotomy

Q38   Pulmonary embolus:

A. Causes 5 deaths per 1000 patients undergoing major surgery
B. Does not arise from a below knee DVT
C. Treatment with systemic heparin should be commenced only after the diagnosis is confirmed with ventilation–perfusion scanning
D. Is a recognised indication for thrombolytic therapy
E. Incidence is decreased in patients with protein C deficiency

Q39   Haemaccel:

A. Is iso-oncotic
B. Has longer half-life *in vivo* than normal saline
C. Has a similar electrolyte content to plasma
D. Is more expensive than Hetastarch
E. Commonly causes anaphylactic reactions
F. Interferes with blood cross-matching

Q40   The acute blood loss of 750 ml in a previously healthy adult results in:

A. Systolic hypotension
B. Tachypnoea > 20/min
C. Slight tachycardia
D. Drowsiness
E. Pale extremities

Q41   Regarding the investigations of a lump in the breast:

A. Fine needle aspiration cytology (FNAC) is highly specific (> 90%)
B. Mammography has a 98% sensitivity
C. Mammography is more sensitive in patients taking HRT
D. Ultrasonography is more useful than mammography in women under the age of 35 years
E. The sensitivity of core biopsy approaches 100%

Q42   During thyroidectomy operation:

A. The right recurrent laryngeal nerve (RLN) is more difficult to locate than the left RLN
B. The right RLN usually passes posterior to the inferior thyroid artery
C. The left RLN usually passes anterior to the inferior thyroid artery
D. The right RLN is located close to the ligaments of Berry
E. The left thyroid lobe is usually larger and located higher than the right lobe

Q43   The following are recognised sites for ectopic parathyroid adenoma:

A. Submandibular gland
B. Posterior triangle of the neck
C. Space of Burns
D. Pericardial cavity
E. Thymus gland

Q44   In primary hyperparathyroidism:

A. Adenomas are multiple in 20% of cases
B. Hyperplasia affects four glands in approximately 15% of cases
C. MRI is the investigation of choice in recurrent cases
D. CT scanning is the most useful localisation technique
E. Oral calcium supplements are contraindicated in all patients

Q45   Urothelial transitional cell carcinoma (TCC):

A. Is commoner in women
B. Incidence is increased among rubber workers
C. Affects the bladder in 95% of cases
D. Is commonly multicentric
E. Frequently presents with polycythaemia

Q46   With respect to tetanus complication a traumatic wound:

A. *Clostridium tetani* travels via the nerves to the anterior horn cells in the spinal cord
B. The tetanospasmin component of the exotoxin acts on synapses to inhibit the normal inhibitory control of motor nerve impulses
C. The diagnosis is usually made relying on microbiological findings
D. The patient should be given large doses of antitoxin intravenously
E. A positive Nagler reaction may identify the presence of *Clostridium tetani* in the wound exudate

Q47   Acute osteomyelitis:

A. Is commonest in children under 10 years old
B. Is caused by *Haemophilus influenzae* in most cases
C. Is rarely associated with positive blood cultures
D. Usually occurs due to a direct spread of bacteria from a neighbouring septic focus or a penetrating wound
E. Is effectively treated with erythromycin and fusidic acid

Q48   Pseudo-membranous colitis:

A. Is a recognised side-effect of clindamycin
B. Is due to colonisation of the colon by *Clostridium perfringens*
C. Procto-sigmoidoscopy is a useful investigation
D. The diagnosis may be made by demonstrating a positive Nagler reaction
E. Is effectively treated with aminoglycosides
F. May be complicated by colonic perforation

Q49   Hepatitis B virus:

A. Contains DNA in its core
B. Carriers rate is approximately 0.1% in south-east Asia
C. E antigen presence in serum indicates increased infectivity
D. Surface antigen antibody usually appears within two weeks of infection
E. Is a recognised cause of hepatic carcinoma

Q50   The identifying criteria of *Staphylococcus aureus* causing a post-operative wound infection include:

A. Coagulase positive
B. Phosphatase negative
C. Fermentation of mannitol
D. Fluorescent greenish appearance of colonies
E. Serology by identification of Lancefield groups

Q51   The following deaths require a coroner's post-mortem:

A. Death due to myocardial infarction during a clinical trial
B. Death due to systemic metastasis of a breast cancer patient undergoing hormonal therapy
C. Death within 24 hours of emergency colectomy for bowel obstruction
D. Death following the insertion of a nasogastric (NG) tube in a head injury patient with a Glasgow coma score of 13 and peri-orbital bruising

Q52   *Streptococcus pyogenes*:

A. Is coagulase negative
B. Produces exotoxin
C. Is typed by phages
D. Lancefield group A, produces β-haemolysis
E. Is a recognised cause of mycotic aneurysms

Q53   The pathophysiological effects of endotoxins include:

A. Inhibition of bradykinin release
B. Release of interleukin 1
C. Inhibition of Hageman factor
D. Activation of the alternative complement pathway
E. Stimulation of platelet aggregation

Q54   Clostridial gas gangrene:

A. Is caused by Gram-positive obligate anaerobes
B. Is a recognised cause of progressive haemolytic anaemia
C. May be treated by placing the patient in a pure oxygen chamber at 13 atmospheres for a few hours daily
D. Pathological and clinical features are mainly due to endotoxins
E. Is relatively common in lower limb amputations for peripheral vascular disease

Q55   Considering wound healing:

A. Fibroblasts are responsible for wound contraction
B. Sutured clean wounds heal by second intention
C. Hyperbaric oxygen enhances the healing of clean surgical wounds
D. Copper deficiency does not affect wound healing
E. There is no inflammatory phase unless the wound is infected

Q56   When the renin-angiotensin-aldosterone system is stimulated by a hypovolaemic shock:

A. Renin converts angiotensin I to angiotensin II
B. Angiotensin II causes vasoconstriction of the efferent glomerular arteriole
C. Angiotensin II stimulates the adrenal medulla to synthesise aldosterone
D. Angiotensin II stimulates the adrenal cortex to increase cortisol production
E. Angiotensin converting enzymes degrade bradykinin

Q57   The following structures lie anterior to the sterno-cleidomastoid muscle:

A. Phrenic nerve
B. External jugular vein
C. Platysma
D. Anterior branch of great auricular nerve
E. Accessory nerve
F. Transverse cervical nerve
G. Omohyoid muscle

Q58   Flail chest:

A. Is characterised by pulsus paradoxus
B. Complicates 20% of significant blunt thoracic trauma
C. Is usually treated with surgical stabilisation of the chest wall
D. Should be managed in an emergency by turning the patient onto the normal side
E. May be treated with epidural narcotics

Q59   A complete division of the femoral nerve results in:

A. Foot drop
B. Paraesthesia of the lateral aspect of the foot
C. Failure of knee extension
D. Sensory loss over the medial part of the lower leg
E. Failure of adduction of the thigh at the hip joint

Q60   Injury to the ulnar nerve at the wrist results in:

A. Wasting of the thenar eminence
B. Clawhand
C. Loss of the pincer-like action of the thumb and index finger
D. Sensory impairment over the palmar surface of the medial one and a half fingers
E. Wasting of the second lumbrical muscle

Theme 1: Mass in the right iliac fossa

A. Appendix mass
B. Tuberculosis
C. Crohn's disease
D. Ulcerative colitis
E. Caecal carcinoma
F. Lymphoma
G. Ectopic kidney

For each type of patients described below, select the most likely treatment from the list of options above. Each option can be used once, more than once or not at all.

Q61   A 20-year-old Somali man presents with a two month history of weight loss, fever and mass in the right iliac fossa (RIF). (Hb: 10 g/dl, WCC: 13 000/mm^3, ESR: 90)

Q62   A 20-year-old Greek man presents with a four month history of weight loss, fever, night sweats and right sided abdominal pain. The pain frequently follows alcohol intake. Clinical examination reveals a mass in the RIF.

Q63   A 70-year-old women presents with nausea, increasing dyspnoea and a mass in the RIF (Hb = 9.8 g/dl, MCV = 65 fl)

Q64   A 25-year-old man is found to have a mobile mass in the RIF during a routine medical examination for insurance purposes

Q65   A 25-year-old man presents with a three-month history of central colicky abdominal pain associated with occasional vomiting and diarrhoea. A barium follow through demonstrates the string sign in the terminal ileum and clinical examination reveals a mass in the RIF

Theme 2: Breast Cancer

A. Wide local excision combined with axillary dissection plus radiotherapy and tamoxifen

B. Simple mastectomy
C. Tamoxifen
D. Radiotherapy
E. Patey's mastectomy
F. Chemotherapy, LHRH analogues and bisphosphonates

For each type of patients described below, select the most likely treatment from the list of options above. Each option can be used once, more than once or not at all.

Q66   A 70-year-old woman presents with a 3 cm lump in the upper outer quadrant of the right breast. The lump does not involve the skin and is mobile. FNAC reveals C5. Mammography shows a speculate lesion corresponding to the lump
Q67   A 40-year-old woman is found to have a widespread micro-calcification during screening mammography. A stereotactic conc biopsy reveals a low grade DCIs
Q68   A 35-year-old woman presents with a 4 cm carcinoma of the left breast and multiple bone metastases in the pelvis
Q69   A 95-year-old woman presents with a locally advanced carcinoma of the left breast

Theme 3: Investigations of the Biliary System

A. ERCP I + sphincterotomy
B. Percutaneous transhepatic cholangiography (PTC)
C. HIDA scan
D. CT scan
E. Oral cholecystogram
F. Serum CA19-9
G. Barium follow through

For each of the patients described below, select the most appropriate investigation from the list of options above. Each option can be used once, more than once or not at all.

Q70   A 59-year-old man presents with obstructive jaundice. USS shows no gallstones. The liver appears normal on USS and the common bile duct (CBD) measures 12 mm in diameter. His past medical history includes partial gastrectomy 15 years ago for peptic ulcer
Q71   A 45-year-old woman presents with upper abdominal pain and obstructive jaundice. The gallbladder is not palpable clinically. USS shows gallstones and a dilated CBD (diameter = 15 mm)
Q72   A 50-year-old obese woman presents with acute upper abdominal pain. Examination demonstrates pyrexia, tachy-

cardia and tenderness in the right upper abdomen. An erect CXR reveals no free intraperitoneal gas. USS fails to confirm the clinical diagnosis of acute cholecystitis

Q73 A 70-year-old woman presents with obstructive jaundice and a palpable gallbladder. USS shows a dilated CBD and enlargement of the pancreatic head. Her past medical history includes polya gastrectomy for a bleeding peptic ulcer

Theme 4: Tumour Markers

A. Carcinoembryonic antigen (CEA)
B. Alpha fetoprotein (AFP)
C. CA19-9
D. Human chorionic gonadotrophic hormone (HCG)
E. CA125
F. Calcitonin
G. Thyroglobulin
H. Prostate specific antigen (PSA)

For each of the tumours below, select the most appropriate serum marker from the list of options above. Each option can be used once, more than once or not at all.

Q74 medullary thyroid cancer
Q75 hepatocellular carcinoma
Q76 rectal carcinoma
Q77 testicular teratoma
Q78 carcinoma of the pancreatic head
Q79 ovarian cancer
Q80 papillary thyroid cancer

Theme 5: Chest Pain in Pregnancy

A. Aortic dissection
B. Massive pulmonary embolus (PE)
C. Pulmonary infarction
D. Myocardial infarction
E. Aortic rupture
F. Hysteria

For each of the clinical scenarios below, select the most appropriate diagnosis from the list of options above. Each option may be used once, more than once or not at all.

Q81 A 30-year-old pregnant women (31 weeks) presents with a severe chest pain of acute onset. There is a family history of ischaemic heart disease. Clinical examination demonstrates dyspnoea, cyanosis, hypotension (90/50 mmHg) and distended neck veins

Q82 A 24-year-old pregnant woman (27 weeks) presents with a six-hour history of pleuritic chest pain and haemoptysis. She has a family history of ischaemic heart disease.

Q83 A tall slim 30-year-old pregnant woman (26 weeks) presents with central chest pain, hypotension (90/40 mmHg) and tachycardia. There is a family history of ischaemic heart disease.

Theme 6: Lump in the Groin

A. Inguinal hernia
B. Femoral hernia
C. Saphenovarix
D. Spigelian hernia
E. Hydrocele

For each of the clinical presentations described below, select the most appropriate diagnosis from the list of options above. Each option may be used once, more than once or not at all.

Q84 A 40-year-old woman presents with a lump in the left groin. The lump is not reducible and lies below an lateral to the pubic tubercle.

Q85 A 40-year-old woman who underwent varicose vein surgery recently presents with a lump in the groin. The lump disappears on lying down and transmits cough impulse. It lies just below the groin crease and medial to the femoral pulse.

Q86 A 60-year-old man presents with a swelling in the groin and scrotum. Clinical examination reveals a scrotal swelling which you can not get above it.

Q87 A 30-year-old man presents with a reducible groin lump lying above and medial to the pubic tubercle

Answers

A1: A(T)   B(T)   C(F)   D(T)   E(F)

In inappropriate ADH secretion, there is dilutional hyponatraemia, decreased plasma osmolality, concentrated urine and continued urinary loss of sodium (> 20 mmol/l). The latter feature is due to the fact that plasma volume is maintained by water retention, thus there is no hypovolaemic stimulus for aldosterone secretion. Aldosterone acts on the distal tubule and collecting duct to retain sodium and excrete potassium.

A2: A(T)   B(F)   C(T)   D(T)   E(F)   F(T)   G(F)

Frusemide increases urinary excretion of potassium. In Addison's disease there is mineralo-corticoid deficiency leading to decreased urinary loss of potassium. Acidosis is associated with hyperkalaemia whereas alkalosis is associated with hypokalaemia. Succinyl choline administration may cause hyperkalaemia.

A3: A(F)   B(F)   C(T)   D(F)   E(F)

The thyrocervical trunk arises from the first part of the subclavian artery. The first part of the subclavian artery also gives rise to the vertebral artery, the costocervical and internal mammary arteries: The deep cervical and superior intercostal arteries are branches of the costocervical artery. The thyrocervical trunk gives rise to the inferior thyroid and suprascapular arteries.

A4: A(T)   B(T)   C(F)   D(T)   E(F)

The median nerve and flexor digitorum superficialis lie deep to the flexor retinaculum, whereas the ulnar artery and nerve lie superficial to it and are therefore vulnerable to injury.

A5: A(T)   B(F)   C(T)   D(T)   E(F)

The vagus nerve passes behind the right main bronchus.

A6: A(F)   B(T)   C(F)   D(T)   E(T)

The fascia transversalis forms the posterior wall of the inguinal canal. The canal transmits the ilio-inguinal nerve. The deep ring moves laterally during growth and development.

A7: A(F) B(F) C(F) D(T) E(T)

Hypoxia impairs the action of the Na^+/K^+ pump leading to Na^+ accumulation in the cell. Oxygen free radicals which contain an odd number of electrons, e.g. O_2^-, are powerful oxidants and capable of damaging cellular DNA. In hydropic degeneration, the cells are waterlogged.

A8: A(F) B(T) C(F) D(F) E(F)

The stylomastoid foramen transmits the VII cranial nerve, the foramen rotundum transmits the maxillary nerve and the foramen lacerum transmits the greater petrosal nerve.

A9: A(F) B(T) C(F) D(F) E(F)

Lysine and proline are incorporated into the protocollagen which is acted upon by protocollagen hydroxylase. The latter requires ascorbic acid (vitamin C) for its action. there is less tissue reaction with synthetic monofilamentous fibres. See Figure 1.

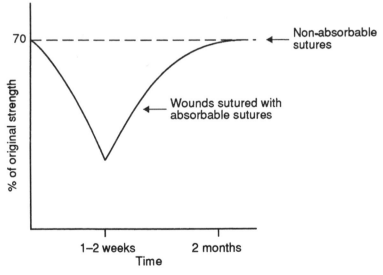

Figure 1

A10: A(T) B(F) C(T) D(T) E(F)

Oncogenes are genes capable of causing cancer. They have been identified in approximately 15% of human cancers. Over expression of oncogenes such as *H-ras* and *K-ras* may lead to gastro-intestinal malignancy, (e.g. pancreas and colon). Other oncogenes include c-erbB2 oncogene (breast cancer) and *c-myc* oncogene. The normal gene is known as a proto-oncogene. Tumour suppressor genes such as p53 represent anti-oncogenes.

A11: A(T) B(F) C(T) D(F) E(F)

Unfractionated heparin has a shorter duration of action than low molecular weight heparin. Heparin anticoagulation is monitored by activated partial thromboplastin time (APTT) whereas INR is used to monitor warfarin anticoagulation. The 5000 units bd regimen is suitable for DVT prophylaxis and not treatment.

A12: A(F) B(T) C(F) D(F) E(F)

The anticoagulation effects of warfarin appear approximately 72 hours after the administration of the first dose. This is because the clotting factors already present in the circulation need to be eliminated. Warfarin has a half-life of about 36 hours and is mainly eliminated by hepatic metabolism. Cimitidine can inhibit the enzyme that metabolises warfarin.

A13: A(F) B(F) C(T) D(F) D(T) F(T)

Familial hypocalciuric hypercalcaemia (FHH) is inherited in an autosomal dominant fashion, therefore the condition can be excluded if both parents are available for blood sampling. The condition is due to avid tubular reabsorption of calcium leading to hypercalcaemia and hypocalciuria. The condition is usually asymptomatic and may present at any age. The kidneys are not usually affected and pancreatitis is a recognised complication.

A14: A(F) B(T) C(T) D(T) E(F)

The pH of stored blood progressively decreases (becomes more acidic). Potassium leaks from damaged cells and blood transfusion can be therefore complicated by hyperkalaemia. Other complications of blood transfusion include hypothermia (due to storage at 4°C), hypocalcaemia (especially if citrate is used for anticoagulation), infections, allergic reactions, DIC, thrombocytopenia and air embolism.

A15: A(T) B(T) C(F) D(T) E(F)

Thrombocytopenia and metabolic acidosis are recognised complications of blood transfusion.

A16: A(F) B(T) C(F) D(T) D(F) F(T)

The normal mammalian cell has 22 pairs of somatic chromosome and one pair of sex chromosomes (XX or XY), therefore the total number of chromosomes is 46.

During the cell cycle (approximately 16 hours), DNA replication occurs during the S-phase and mitosis occurs during the M-phase. Chromosomes are not easily visible by light microscopy during the interphase. Chromosome condensation starts during mitosis (prophase, metaphase and telophase). Gametes are haploid (23 chromosomes) whereas fertilised eggs are diploid (46 chromosomes). The nucleus has an outer membrane (endoplasmic reticulum) and an inner membrane. The latter contains pores for exchange with the cytoplasm.

A17: A(T) B(T) C(T) D(F) E(F)
Splenectomy and sarcoidosis are associated with thrombocytosis.

A18: A(F) B(F) C(T) D(F) E(T)
PT is usually normal in patients with haemophilia A due to deficiency of factor VIIIC.

20% of normal factor VIII activity is required for minor bleeds. Major surgery requires 60%. Factor VIII injections have a half-life of 12 hours, therefore administration is twice daily.

A19: A(T) B(T) C(T) D(T) E(F)
The endotoxin (a lipopolysaccharide) stimulates immunocytes to release cytokines such as IL-1 and TNF-α. The cytokines influence thermoregulation, endocrine function and metabolic responses. They also mediate the inflammatory responses in shock which is responsible for many of the clinical consequences, e.g. ARDS, interstitial oedema, etc. TNF-α and IL-1 stimulate the cyclo-oxygenase factor and nitric oxide synthase. Gastrointestinal haemorrhage may be secondary to uraemia and DIC. Interstitial oedema results from increased vascular permeability. Acute tubular necrosis and renal failure are also recognised consequences. Septic shock may lead to multiple organ failure.

A20: A(F) B(F) C(T) D(F) E(T)
Polyester (Dacron), polyamide (nylon) and polypropylene (Prolene) are synthetic non-absorbable sutures. Polydioannone and polyglycolic acid are also known as PDS and Dexon respectively.

A21: A(F) B(F) C(F) D(T) E(T)
Lignocaine inhibits the rapid inflow of Na^+ into excitable cells by displacing Ca^{2+} from its sites on membrane phospholipids. Lignocaine is a weak base. The local tissue acidosis of inflammation shifts the drug towards the ionised lipid-insoluble form which is less

effective. The maximal safe dose is 3 mg per kg. This can be doubled with the addition of adrenaline.

A22: A(F) B(T) C(F) D(T) E(F)

Pulse oximetry uses two wavelengths of light. Beer's law indicates that the concentration of a solute can be determined by light absorption. Finger probes are less rapid but more precise than ear probes. Nail polish tends to underestimate the oxygen saturation reading of pulse oximeters.

A23: A(F) B(T) C(F) D(F) E(F)

Autoclaving utilises moist steam at 121°C and a pressure of 15 lb/in². The procedure requires 15–20 min for sterilisation. Glassware is usually sterilised by dry heat at 180°C.

A24: A(T) B(T) C(F) D(F) E(T)

Surgical diathermy uses an electrosurgical unit that converts 50 Hz a.c. (hazardous) into 50,000 Hz a.c. (safe). The bipolar type heats only tissue held between the diathermy forceps thus causing less surrounding tissue damage than the monopolar type. The latter is avoided in circumcision, when operating near important nerves and in the presence of cardiac pacemakers. The monopolar diathermy plate should be applied close to the surgical field in order to reduce the amount of tissue that the current passes through to reach the plate.

A25: A(F) B(F) C(T) D(F) E(T)

Screening mammography has been shown to reduce breast cancer mortality in women over the age of 50 years. Young women tend to have dense breasts which are difficult to assess with mammography. Mammography may reveal microcalcifications, speculate masses, stellate lesions and architectural distortions in malignancy. Round microcalcification is usually benign. The radiation dose of mammography is too small to increase the risk of breast cancer.

A26: A(T) B(F) C(F) D(T) E(T)

Level I axillary nodes lie lateral to the pectoralis minor muscle, level II nodes lie behind the muscle and level III nodes lie medial to the muscle. Axillary clearance implies removal of all three levels. The sentinel node status correlates well with the axillary basin status. It can be identified using blue dyes or radioisotopes.

A27: A(T) B(F) C(T) D(T) E(F)

Screening mammography has reduced breast cancer mortality by
25% in women over the age of 50 years. In premenopausal
patients, cytotoxic chemotherapy and oophorectomy (surgical or
chemical) has been shown to reduce mortality. In post menopausal
patients, tamoxifen and chemotherapy can reduce mortality. Recent
studies have demonstrated that post mastectomy radiotherapy can
reduce mortality in premenopausal women with node positive
cancer. Tamoxifen reduces mortality in ER-positive patients regard-
less of age.

A28: A(F) B(T) C(F) D(T) E(T)

Posterior shoulder dislocation which is frequently seen in epileptics,
is much less common than anterior shoulder dislocation. In anterior
dislocation, there is flattening of the shoulder contour and the arm
is held in the abduction position (30%). Axillary nerve palsy may
cause deltoid muscle atrophy and paraesthesia in the upper arm.
Treatment methods include Kocher's and the hippocratic man-
oeuvres.

A29: A(T) B(F) C(F) D(T) E(F)

The causes of carpal tunnel syndrome (CTS) include pregnancy,
R.A., hyperthyroidism, osteoarthritis and fractures in the region of
the wrist. The syndrome results from compression of the median
nerve in the tunnel under the flexor retinaculum. The nerve
supplies motor innervation to the abductor pollicis bresis muscle.
The differential diagnosis of CTS includes cervical rib which may
produce similar symptoms. The CTS is treated by dividing the flexor
retinaculum. The division may be performed endoscopically.

A30: A(T) B(T) C(F) D(F) E(F)

Factors favouring good prognosis in cutaneous melanoma include
female sex, low Breslow's thickness, superficial Clark's level,
peripheral location and younger age.

A31: A(F) B(T) C(T) D(F) E(F)

Polycythaemia and states of decreased 2,3-DPG shift the curve to
the left. Shift to the right implies that the haemoglobin gives up
oxygen readily in peripheral tissues. This is desirable in anaemia,
respiratory acidosis and pyrexia.

A32: A(T) B(F) C(F) D(T) E(F)

Metabolic acidosis is characterised by a low arterial pH and a reduced serum bicarbonate (HCO_3^-). The causes include hypovolaemia, diabetic ketoacidosis, ingestion of alcohol and salicylates, septicaemia renal failure, tissue necrosis, loss of HCO_3^- and massive blood transfusions. HCO_3^- is the main extracellular buffer whereas proteins and phosphates represent the main intracellular buffers. Compensation occurs by an increase in alveolar ventilation (respiratory) and an increase in H^+ excretion and HCO_3^- reabsorption by the kidneys (renal). Treatment is aimed at correcting cause. This often entails intravenous fluid replacement.

A33: A(T) B(F) C(T) D(F) E(T)
Captopril (ACE inhibitor) and Spironolactone (aldosterone antagonist) may cause hyperkalaemia. In Conn's syndrome, there is excessive production of aldosterone which causes sodium retention and potassium loss. In diabetes insipidus, there is haemodilation due to water retention caused by excessive ADH. Excessive loss of potassium-rich secretion by villous adenoma can lead to hypokalaemia.

A34: A(F) B(T) C(F) D(F) E(F)
Iron is primarily absorbed in the duodenum and jejunum. Gastric acid tends to break insoluble iron complexes and thus facilitates iron absorption. Ascorbic acid reduces Fe^{3+} to Fe^{2+} thus increasing iron absorption. Absorbed iron binds to apoferritin in enterocytes to firm ferritin. It is transported into the plasma by transferrin (β-globulin). In iron deficiency, there is a decrease in serum iron and ferritin levels. Total iron binding capacity (TIBC) is increased in iron deficiency states.

A35: A(T) B(F) C(F) D(T) E(T) F(T) G(T)
Cardiac tamponade is characterised by hypotension, muffled heart sounds and raised JVP (Beck's triad). Pericardiocentesis can be helpful in confirming the diagnosis of two-dimensional echocardiography. It is not immediately available, however thoracotomy is usually required in trauma patients with cardiac tamponade. Kussmaul's sign refers to a rise in JVP on inspiration.

A36: A(F) B(T) C(T) D(F) E(T)
In massive abdominal haemorrhage, aortic cross clamping and intra aortic transfusion facilitates preferential perfusion of the brain and myocardium and arrests abdominal bleeding. Elective thoracotomy is indicated if the initial chest drain insertion reveals > 1500 ml of blood immediately or if 250 ml is drained in three consecutive hours

with no decreasing rate. Other indications for elective thoracotomy include cardiac tamponade, massive air leak, mediastinal wounds, chest wall defects, clotted haemothorax and empyema.

A37: A(T) B(F) C(F) D(T) E(F)

Preoperative breathing exercises and stopping smoking reduce the risk of postoperative pulmonary atelectasis. Postoperative chest physiotherapy is the mainstay of treatment. Humidified oxygen and antibiotics are also used in treatment. Flexible bronchoscopy is occasionally used to remove a mucus plug causing collapse of a large pulmonary segment.

A38: A(T) B(F) C(F) D(T) E(F)

Systemic heparin therapy should be commenced once the diagnosis is suspected. Approximately 30% of calf DVTs propagate and 20% of these propagations occur above the knee increasing the risk of pulmonary thromboembolisms. Thrombophilic conditions such as protein C deficiency, protein S deficiency, factor V Laiden, anti-thrombin deficiency and phospholipid syndrome are associated with an increased risk of PE.

A39: A(T) B(T) C(F) D(F) E(F)

Polygelatins including Haemaccel and Gelfusion have a half-life *in vitro* of 6–8 hours. They are cheap and suitable for replacing blood loss with or without blood transfusion to maintain a packed cell volume of 30%. Polygelatins are cheaper than Hetastarch and have a low incidence of anaphylactic reactions.

A40: A(F) B(F) C(T) D(F) E(F)

Hypovolaemic shock can be classified into four classes according to blood loss. The percentage blood loss is < 15% in class I, 15–30% in class II, 30–40% in class III and > 40% in class IV. In previously healthy adults, systolic blood pressure is often preserved despite losing 1.5–2.0 litres of blood due to the effective response of sympathetic stimulation. Class I patients usually have no symptoms. Blood pressure falls in class III and IV patients.

A41: A(T) B(F) C(F) D(T) E(F)

FNAC is more sensitive than core biopsy in establishing the diagnosis of breast cancer. However, it cannot distinguish between invasive and non-invasive breast cancer. FNAC is highly specific in the hands of experienced cytologists.

The sensitivity of mammography is approximately 85%. It is less useful in young women who tend to have dense breasts. In women ≤35 years, USS is more informative. HRT tends to increase breast density thus reducing the sensitivity of mammography.

A42: A(T) B(F) C(F) D(T) E(F)

The right RLN is more difficult to locate than the left RLN. The former usually passes anterior to the inferior thyroid artery whereas the latter usually passes posterior to the artery. The right RLN may be aberrant and arise high from the vagus. Ligaments of Berry bind the deep surface of the thyroid to the upper lateral trachea and cricoid cartilage. The right thyroid lobe is slightly larger and placed higher than the left, hence mobilisation of the right upper pole may be difficult.

A43: A(T) B(T) C(T) D(T) E(T)

If thorough neck exploration fails to reveal an expected parathyroid adenoma, then further investigations and mediastinal exploration are indicated. Selective venous sampling, subtraction imaging, real-time ultrasonography, CT and MRI are useful investigations. Intra-operative venous sampling can also be performed, but this facility is not widely available.

A44: A(F) B(T) C(F) D(F) E(F)

An American series reported multiple adenomas in 2.5% of cases and four-gland hyperplasia in 15% of cases. Selective venous sampling and subtraction imaging are useful localisation techniques but the Sestamibi scan is the most accurate localisation modality. MRI is currently under investigation but there is no evidence that it is superior to CT scanning. Expert neck ultrasonography is a useful pre-operative investigation. Patients with severe bony changes may benefit from oral calcium and vitamin D unless serum calcium is grossly elevated.

A45: A(F) B(T) C(T) D(T) E(F)

The incidence of urothelial carcinoma is 17 per 10^5 per annum. The male to female ratio is 3:1. The risk factors including smoking and occupational hazards (rubber, aniline dye and plastics). Haematuria is the commonest symptom. The investigations of patients with haematuria should include urine microscopy and culture, urine cytology, intravenous urography and cystoscopy.

Intravesical mitomycin and BCG are used in the treatment of superficial TCC and carcinoma *in situ* of the bladder. Radical radio-therapy is indicated for invasive TCC in the elderly and for palliation.

A46: A(F) B(T) C(F) D(T) E(F)

Clostridium tetani does not spread beyond the wound, but the exotoxin travels via the nerves to the anterior horn cells of the spinal cord. The diagnosis is usually made on clinical grounds. Nagler reaction is used in the identification of *Clostridium perfringens*.

A47: A(T) B(F) C(F) D(F) E(T)

Acute osteomyelitis is caused by *Staphylococcus aureus* in most cases and blood cultures are positive in a significant proportion of cases. Bacteria usually reach the bone via the blood stream.

A48: A(T) B(F) C(T) D(F) E(F) F(T)

Pseudomembranous colitis is caused by *Clostridium difficile* and associated with the use of antibiotics sigmoidoscopy may reveal pseudomembranous plaques which can be biopsied. The condition is treated by metronidazole or vancomycin. Clostridia are generally resistant to aminoglycosides.

A49: A(T) B(F) C(T) D(F) E(T)

The carrier's rate in South East Asia is approximately 10% (0.1% in the U.K.). The presence of e-antigen and DNA polymerase in serum indicates increased infectivity. Surface antigen antibodies appear late and indicate immunity. The incidence of hepatic carcinoma is increased by 300-fold in infected patients.

A50: A(T) B(F) C(T) D(F) E(F)

S. aureus colonies are typically golden yellow and phosphatase positive. Lancefield classification applies to streptococci whereas phage typing applies to *S. aureus*.

A51: A(T) B(F) C(T) D(T)

Caution should be exercised when passing an NG tube in patients with suspected basal skull fractures as the tube can easily penetrate the intracranial cavity.

A52: A(F) B(T) C(F) D(T) E(T)

S. pyogenes is coagulase positive. Phage typing applies to staphylococci.

A53: A(F) B(T) C(F) D(T) E(T)

Cytokines such as interleukin 1 and tumour necrosis factor alpha mediate the clinical manifestations of septic shock. Hageman factor is stimulated and bradykinin levels are increased. The latter causes vasodilation and hypotension.

A54: A(T) B(T) C(F) D(F) E(T)
Exotoxins especially α-toxin (lecithinase) are primarily responsible for the clinical manifestations of clostridial sepsis. In hyperbaric oxygen therapy, the pressure does not usually exceed three atmos–pheres.

A55: A(T) B(F) C(F) D(F) E(F)
Clean wounds which are sutured heal by first intention. Wounds which are unsutured heal more slowly by second intention which is characterised by the formation of granulation tissue. Hyperbaric oxygen has a role in the management of wounds infected by anaerobic bacteria such as clostridial gas gangrene. Copper deficiency can delay would healing. There is a mild inflammatory phase (in 24 hours) in all healing wounds.

A56: A(F) B(T) C(F) D(F) E(T)
Renin converts angiotensinogen to angiotensin I. Angiotensin converting enzymes convert angiotensin I to angiotensin II in the lungs. Angiotensin II stimulates the adrenal cortex to secrete aldosterone and causes vasoconstriction. Bradykinin has vasodila-ting effects.

A57: A(F) B(T) C(T) D(T) E(F) F(T) G(F)
The phrenic nerve, the accessory nerve, and the omohyoid muscle lie deep to the sternocleido mastoid muscle.

A58: A(F) B(T) C(F) D(F) E(T)
Paradoxical chest movement is characteristic of flail chest. Flail chest is treated mainly by ventilation, analgesia and physiotherapy. The flail segment may be stabilised by turning the patient onto the affected side.

A59: A(F) B(F) C(T) D(T) E(F)
Common peroneal nerve injury causes foot drop and sensory impairment on the lateral aspect of the foot. Thigh adductors are supplied by the obturator nerve.

A60: A(F) B(T) C(F) D(T) E(F)
Wasting of the thenar eminence and the first and second lumbrical muscles are features of medial nerve palsy. The pincer action of the thumb and index fingers is only slightly impaired due to paralysis of the adductor pollicis muscle.

A61: B
The origin of this patient and clinical history including elevated ESR makes TB most likely.

A62: F
The Mediterranean origin and alcohol-associated pain suggest lymphoma.

A63: E
The microcytic anaemia and age of patient makes caecal carcinoma the most likely diagnosis.

A64: G

A65: C

A66: A

A67: B
Axillary clearance is not indicated in low grade DCIS. The tumour seems to be widespread on mammography therefore mastectomy is indicated. Axillary sampling may be performed.

A68: F
High-dose chemotherapy, including adriamycin and Taxol, is indicated in this young patient. Peripheral stem cell and antologous bone marrow support may be necessary. LHRH analogues and biphosphates are also indicated.

A69: C
In this frail patient, tamoxifen alone may suffice especially if the tumour is ER-positive.

A70: B
ERCP is not the most appropriate option in this patient in view of the gastrectomy in the past. PTC is a good imaging modality in this patient.

A71: A
ERCP will outline the CBD and reveal any obstructive gallstones. Sphincterotomy and removal of the CBD stones may be performed at the time of ERCP.

A72: C
HIDA scan may support the clinical diagnosis of acute cholecystitis. Inflamed gallbladder is not usually functional and will not concentrate the radioactive contrast.

A73: D
CT scanning in this patient may reveal a pancreatic tumour causing the jaundice.

A74: F

A75: B

A76: A

A77: B

A78: C

A79: E

A80: G

A81: B
The cyanosis, hypotension and distended neck veins suggest that massive PE is more likely than pulmonary infarction.

A82: C

A83: A
The physical description of the patient suggests Marfan's syndrome which is associated with increased incidence of aortic dissection.

A84: B
The patient's sex, the lump location (below and lateral to the pubic tubercle) and the fact that the lump is not reducible make femoral hernia the most likely diagnosis.

A85: C

A86: A
This patient seems to have an inguinoscrotal hernia.

A87: A

Core Modules Paper B

Questions

Q1 In burns patients, the following are recognised features:

A. Cystinuria
B. Myoglobinuria
C. Gastric ulcers
D. Hyperkalaemia
E. Metabolic alkalosis

Q2 During axillary dissection, the surgeon finds that:

A. The nerve to the latissimus dorsi runs with the vascular pedicle of the subscapularis
B. The long thoracic nerve is closely applied to the chest wall at the posterior-medial aspect of the dissection
C. The pectoralis minor muscle is inserted into the acromion
D. Level III axillary nodes lie lateral to the pectoralis minor muscle
E. The teres major, subscapularis and latissimus dorsi muscles form the posterior axillary wall

Q3 With respect to the blood supply to the femoral head:

A. The obturator artery supplies the head via a branch which ascends through the femoral neck
B. The blood supply from the branch of the obturator artery is the most important item
C. The medial circumflex femoral artery supplies the head via branches that ascend along the neck deep to the synovial membrane
D. Extracapsular fractures of the femoral neck severely damage the blood supply to the head
E. Displaced subcapital fractures of the femoral head seriously damage the blood supply to the head

**Q4   The long saphenous vein usually receives the follow-
         ing tributaries in the femoral triangle:**

A. The superficial epigastric vein
B. The deep circumflex iliac vein
C. The deep external pudendal vein
D. The lateral accessory vein
E. The superficial circumflex iliac vein

Q5   Regarding peripheral nerve injuries:

A. Transient impairment of conduction is known as neuropraxia
B. A crushing injury is most likely to be neurotmesis
C. Primary nerve repair is desirable for an inadvertent nerve section
   during a clean surgical operation
D. The axon grows at 1mm/day after nerve section
E. The distal axon undergoes Wallerian degeneration

**Q6   With respect to the gallbladder and common bile duct
         (CBD):**

A. The cystic artery branches from the right hepatic artery and lies
   most commonly between the cystic duct and liver
B. The right hepatic duct rarely enters the gallbladder near its
   junction with the cystic duct
C. The internal diameter of a normal CBD is about 12mm on
   ultrasonography
D. The wall of the supraduodenal part of the CBD has a venous
   plexus which can be seen at operation
E. The incidence of CBD injury is higher for laparoscopic
   cholecystectomy than for open cholecystectomy
F. The inflamed gall bladder appears as a hot spot on the HIDA scan

Q7   In the root of the neck:

A. The subclavian vein crosses the first rib posterior to scalenus
   anterior
B. The phrenic nerve descends anterior to scalenus anterior
C. The cervical dome of pleura lies behind scalenus medius
D. The stellate ganglion lies at the level of C7 vertebra
E. The subclavian artery crosses the first rib anterior to scalenus
   anterior

Q8   With respect to fracture healing:

A. The cells of the deeper layer of the periosteum have osteogenic potential
B. The pH of the uniting fracture starts decreasing after about 10 days
C. The bone ends show osteoporosis in the early stages of fracture healing
D. Hyperparathyroidism impairs fracture healing
E. Globules of fat may enter disrupted vascular spaces and become embolic

Q9   Obstructive jaundice usually:

A. Reduces vitamin D absorption from the gastrointestinal tract
B. Reduces prothrombin time (PT)
C. Increases urinary excretion of urobilinogen
D. Causes dark urine and pale stools
E. Elevates the serum level of alkaline phosphatase
F. Causes steatorrhoea

Q10   The following are commoner in Crohn's disease than in ulcerative colitis:

A. Crypt abscesses in the bowel mucosa
B. Pseudopolyps in the bowel lumen
C. The development of carcinoma as a complication
D. Bowel obstruction as a complication
E. Involvement of the submucosa and deeper layers

Q11   Ductal carcinoma *in situ* (DCIS) of the breast:

A. Presents as a palpable mass in approximately 70% of cases
B. Is associated with positive axillary nodes in 20% of cases
C. Is characterised by microcalcification on the mammogram
D. Of the comedo type has a better prognosis than the solid type
E. May become invasive if left untreated

Q12 **The following are recognised features of strenuous exercise:**

A. Increased serum lactate
B. Increased stroke volume
C. Increased blood pH
D. Hypertension
E. Reduced serum creatinine phosphate kinase (CPK)

Q13 **Cholinergic impulses in the autonomic nervous system produce:**

A. A decrease in atrial contractility
B. Detrusor muscle relaxation
C. Ciliary muscle contraction
D. Gallbladder relaxation
E. Ejaculation
F. Increased intestinal motility

Q14 **The following factors stimulate gastrin secretion:**

A. Increased vagal activity
B. Hypercalcaemia
C. Increased gastric acidity
D. Secretin
E. A protein meal

Q15 **Figure 2 shows the various parts of the electrocardiogram. The following statements are correct:**

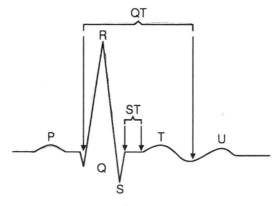

Figure 2

A. Opening of the aortic valve coincides with the P wave
B. Isovolumetric contraction occurs during the P wave
C. During the ST segments all parts of ventricles have been depolarised
D. The QT interval may be prolonged in hypokalaemia
E. During the T wave, the tricuspid valve is normally closed
F. The first heart sound occurs just after the QRS complex

Q16   The following may reduce intracranial pressure (ICP):

A. Hypoventilation
B. Intravenous mannitol
C. The administration of atracurium
D. The administration of hyperbaric oxygen
E. Positioning the patient in the head down position

Q17   The following factors impair wound healing:

A. Corticosteroids
B. Mild anaemia
C. Hypoalbuminaemia
D. Haematoma formation
E. Ultraviolet light
F. Jaundice

Q18   Primary hyperparathyroidism:

A. Is most common in premenopausal women
B. Is caused by hyperplasia of parathyroid glands in most cases
C. May be complicated by hypertension
D. Is characterised by elevated serum phosphate
E. Causes bone demineralisation
F. Impairs fracture healing
G. Rarely requires surgical treatment

Q19   When designing a screening test for malignancy:

A. The tumour should be of the anaplastic type
B. The tumour should have a short latency
C. The test should be more specific than sensitive
D. The test should be highly sensitive
E. The test should have a low inter-observer error

Q20   The consequences of chronic liver disease include:

A. Hypergammaglobulinaemia
B. Hypoalbuminaemia
C. Encephalopathy
D. Low plasma levels of factor VIII
E. Prolonged prothrombin time

Q21   Fat embolus:

A. May arise from plasma lipids
B. Usually occurs about 10 days after major fractures
C. Passes through the pulmonary filter to the cerebral circulation in most cases
D. Is associated with increased plasma lipase levels in about 75% of cases
E. Commonly causes pyoderma gangrenosum

Q22   The causes of hypocalcaemia include:

A. Pseudohypoparathyroidism
B. Acute pancreatitis
C. Milk-alkali syndrome
D. Sarcoidosis
E. Magnesium deficiency

Q23   The following are recognised causes of hypercalcaemia:

A. Bronchial carcinoma
B. Thiazide diuretics
C. Bisphosphonates
D. Thyrotoxicosis
E. Pseudohypoparathyroidism

Q24   Failure to excrete a water load (1 litre taken orally) is a recognised feature of:

A. Bronchial carcinoma
B. Loss of hypothalamic osmotic receptors
C. Cranial diabetes insipidus
D. Hepatic failure
E. Hyperglycaemia

Q25 Hyperacute renal transplant rejection:

A. Is cell mediated
B. Usually occurs within hours of transplantation
C. Responds to corticosteroids
D. Incidence is decreased by the use of cyclosporin A
E. Is best treated by removal of transplant

Q26 With reference to complications of total hip arthroplasty, the following are true:

A. Hip dislocation occurs in approximately 15% of cases
B. Sciatic nerve injury is a recognised complication
C. The incidence of loosening is approximately 35% at 15-year follow up
D. There is no evidence that prophylactic antibiotics reduce infection rate
E. Unfractionated heparin is more effective in preventing DVT than low molecular weight heparin

Q27 The following are recognised complications of deep venous thrombosis (DVT):

A. Milroy's disease
B. Phlegmasia cerula dolens
C. Cystic hygroma of the lower limb
D. Phlegmasia alba dolens
E. Venous claudication

Q28 In compartment syndrome:

A. Nerves can survive ischaemia for 8 hours
B. Muscle can survive ischaemia for 8 hours
C. The presence of distal peripheral pulses excludes the syndrome
D. The intracompartmental pressure usually exceeds 30 mmHg
E. Fasciotomy is contraindicated

Q29 The following are recognised complications of trache-ostomy:

A. Surgical emphysema
B. Pneumonia
C. Air embolism
D. Haemorrhage
E. Subglottic stenosis

Q30 Adenomatous polyposis coli 'APC' syndrome:

A. Is inherited as an autosomal dominant disorder
B. Is due to a genetic defect located on the short arm of chromosome 5
C. Patients typically have more than 100 colorectal polyps
D. Usually presents in the sixth decade
E. Is an indication for family screening
F. Mainstay of management is regular surveillance of the colon

Q31 The following factors predict a good prognosis in malignant melanoma:

A. Male sex
B. Low Breslow thickness
C. The presence of ulceration
D. Older age
E. A mucosal primary site

Q32 Cyclophosphamide:

A. Is inactive until is hydroxylated by hepatic enzymes
B. Metabolites include MESNA
C. Binds to the protein tubulin, thereby preventing the formation of microtubules
D. Is well absorbed orally
E. Is less myelotoxic than ifosfamide
F. May cause gonadal damage

Q33 The following are recognised risk factors for carcinoma of the colon:

A. Melanosis coli
B. Gardner's syndrome
C. Crohn's disease
D. Diverticular disease
E. Colonic angiodysplasia
F. Ureterosigmoidostomy

Q34   Colorectal carcinoma:

A. Has a higher incidence in third world countries
B. Arising in the right colon usually presents with bowel obstruction
C. Commonest organ of metastasis is the liver
D. Screening methods include faecal occult blood (FOB) testing
E. Serum marker is alpha-fetoprotein
F. Is relatively sensitive to 5-fluorouracil

Q35   Osteogenic sarcoma:

A. Most commonly affects the metaphysis of the femur
B. Has two peaks of incidence
C. Develops in 35% of patients with Paget's disease of the bone
D. Radiological features include Codman's triangle
E. Of the limb, is treated by amputation in most cases
F. Commonest site of metastases is the liver
G. Overall 5-year survival rate exceeds 50%

Q36   With reference to the blood supply of the colorectum, the following statements are correct:

A. The left colic artery arises from the superior mesenteric (SMA)
B. The middle colic artery arises from the inferior mesenteric artery (IMA)
C. The IMA communicates with the SMA via the marginal artery of Drummond
D. The hepatic flexure is mainly supplied by branches of the SMA
E. The middle rectal artery arises from the external iliac artery
F. The splenic flexure is mainly supplied by the left colic artery

Q37   Gastrointestinal lymphoma:

A. Is a recognised complication of dermatitis herpetiformis
B. Peak incidence occurs during the third decade
C. Associated with Coeliac disease is usually B cell lymphoma
D. Commonest site is the terminal ileum
E. May present with peritonitis
F. Associated with extra abdominal lymph node metastases, should be treated by surgical resection
G. Is radiosensitive

Q38 Recognised risk factors for oesophageal carcinoma include:

A. Barrett's oesophagus
B. Diverticular disease of the oesophagus
C. Zinc deficiency
D. Regular intake of vitamin C supplements
E. Ulcerative colitis
F. Achalasia
G. Alpha-chain disease
H. *Helicobacter pylori* infection

Q39 The consequences of raised intracranial pressure (ICP) include:

A. Tachycardia
B. Papilloedema
C. Systemic hypertension
D. Midbrain haemorrhage
E. Vomiting
F. Battle's sign
G. False-localising signs

Q40 With reference to pyogenic infections of the flexor synovial sheath of the index finger:

A. The index finger is usually held in flexion
B. The absence of overlying oedema and erythema excludes the diagnosis
C. Proximal spread of infection is common
D. Intravenous antibiotics is the mainstay of management
E. Fixed flexion deformity is a recognised complication

Q41 Recognised complications of acute pancreatitis include:

A. Pleural effusion
B. Upper gastrointestinal haemorrage
C. Adult respiratory distress syndrome
D. Hypertrophic obstructive cardiomyopathy
E. Acanthosis nigricans

Q42   When performing an appendicectomy through the gridiron incision the surgeon will encounter:

A. The fibres of the external oblique muscle lying perpendicular to the line of incision
B. The fibres of the internal oblique and transversus abdominis lying almost in a transverse direction
C. Scarpa's fascia deep to the external oblique aponeurosis
D. The trasversalis fascia fused to the peritoneum
E. Numerous communications between the appendicular artery and the ileal artcries

Q43   The great saphenous vein:

A. Passes behind the medial malleolus
B. Joins the femoral vein about 3.5 cm below and lateral to the pubic tubercle
C. Usually lies behind the superficial external pudendal artery
D. Receives fewer tributaries than the femoral vein at the level of the saphenous opening
E. Has more deep perforators below the knee than in the thigh

Q44   The following myocutaneous flaps (MF) and vascular pedicles are correctly paired:

A. Latissimus dorsi MF – subscapular artery
B. Transverse rectus abdominis MF – superficial circumflex iliac artery
C. Tensor fascia lata MF – transverse branch of the lateral femoral circumflex artery
D. Gracilis MF – lateral femoral circumflex artery
E. Pectoralis major MF – thoracoacromial artery

Q45   When exposing the popliteal artery as part of an exploration of the popliteal fossa the surgeon will find the following relations:

A. The tibial nerve lies deep to the artery
B. The popliteal vein lies between the popliteal artery and tibial nerve
C. The artery lies on the popliteal ligament of the knee joint
D. The tendon of semitendinosus lies lateral to the artery
E. The peroneal nerve lies lateral to the artery

Q46 Renal injuries:

A. Are caused by penetrating trauma in 85% of cases
B. Are managed conservatively in most cases
C. May cause hypertension
D. Associated with macroscopic haematuria should be investigated with intravenous urography (IVU)
E. Should be investigated with angiography if there is frank haematuria
F. Are more accurately assessed by ultrasound than CT scanning

Q47 Diagnostic peritoneal lavage (DPL) in a trauma patient:

A. Is relatively contraindicated in pregnancy
B. Should be performed if there is unexplained shock
C. Is regarded as positive if the fluid red blood cell (RBC) count is > 10 000/mm^3
D. Is regarded as positive if the fluid amylase level is 30 units
E. Has a high false-positive rate

Q48 The indications for thoracotomy following thoracic trauma include:

A. Haemothorax with initial drainage of 450 ml of blood
B. Haemothorax with bleeding at a rate of 200 ml/hour for four consecutive hours
C. Empyema
D. Cardiac tamponade
E. Flail chest with $PO_2 = 9$ kPa and $PCO_2 = 7$ kPa

Q49 The acute blood loss of 1.5 litres leads to a decrease in:

A. The rate of oxygen extraction by peripheral tissues
B. The firing rate of carotid and aortic baroreceptors
C. Renin secretion
D. Peripheral vascular tone
E. Cardiac output

Q50 The expert witness in a medial litigation case:

A. Has a prime duty toward the court rather than his/her client
B. Can not be sued
C. Should not communicate with the expert witness of the other side prior to court hearing
D. Must be an NHS consultant
E. Concerning causation rather than negligence should be a specialist in the medical field in which the case arose

Q51   The spinothalamic tracts of the spinal cord transmit the following sensory modalities:

A. Pain
B. Two-point discrimination
C. Joint position
D. Temperature
E. Vibration

Q52   During the surgical approach to the submandibular gland, the following structures are found to lie superficial to the superficial part of the submandibular gland:

A. Hypoglossal nerve
B. Platysma
C. Facial vein
D. Cervical branch of facial nerve
E. Superior laryngeal nerve
F. Digastric muscle
G. Lingual nerve

Q53   The brain:

A. Receives 5% of the cardiac output
B. Blood flow to the brain is 800 ml/min
C. Intracranial pressure (ICP) is normally 0–10 mmHg
D. Intracranial pressure is directly proportional to the volume of skull contents
E. Compensates for initial rise in ICP by losing CSF in the lumbar thecal sac

Q54   Cervical spine radiographs:

A. Normally show a 6 mm atlanto-odontoid gap in adults
B. Open mouth odontoid views may show Jefferson fracture
C. Should be taken in a multiple trauma patient
D. Swimmers view allows assessment of upper cervical vertebrae
E. Showing displacement > 50% of vertebral width usually indicate bilateral facet dislocation

Q55   Cerebral blood flow:

A. Accounts for about 15% of the cardiac output
B. Is decreased by hypocapnia
C. Is decreased by hypoxia
D. Is mainly controlled by sympathetic and parasympathetic mechanisms
E. Is increased by isoflurane in general anaesthesia

Q56   Consider the following head CT scan of a trauma
patient (Figure 1). The statements below are correct:

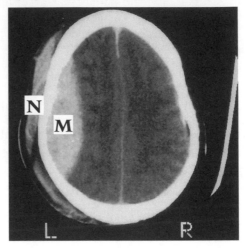

Figure 3

A. M represents an extradural haematoma
B. N represents soft tissue swelling
C. A lumbar puncture is contraindicated in this patient
D. Hyperventilation should be avoided during the initial management
E. Urgent neurosurgery is indicated
F. 50% Mannitol solution should be given intravenously (10g/kg)

Q57   The clinical signs of pericardial tamponade include:

A. Loud heart sounds
B. Hypotension
C. Pulsus paradoxicus
D. Tachycardia
E. Reduced jugular venous pressure (JVP)

Q58   The clinical signs of spinal cord injury include:

A. Priapism
B. Decreased anal sphincter tone
C. Hypertension
D. Cullen's sign
E. Urinary retention
F. Tachycardia (assuming no significant hypovolaemia)
G. Sensory ataxia

Q59   During intubation of a patient with a head injury:

A. It should be assumed that the patient has a cervical spine fracture
B. The intubating doctor must clearly visualise the vocal cords prior to intubation
C. Pressure on the cricoid cartilage must be avoided
D. A nasogastric tube should be passed in all cases
E. Tracheostomy is necessary if the intubation cannot be performed

Q60   In the initial management of the burned patient:

A. Phenol burns should be placed under running water
B. IV fluid replacement is necessary in burns over > 15% of the body surface area
C. Tetanus prophylaxis is not necessary
D. Blood transfusion should be given if haematocrit falls to 35%
E. Systemic antibiotics should be used routinely

Theme 1: Fluid Resuscitation

A. Blood transfusion
B. Haemaccel (polygelatin)
C. Normal saline
D. 5% dextrose
E. Polygelatin plus blood

For each episode of hypovolaemia described below, select the most appropriate fluid for resuscitation from the list of options above. Each option may be used once, more than once, or not at all.

Q61   Acute blood loss of 900 ml in an 84-year-old woman (systolic BP = 90 mmHg

Q62   An insulin-dependent diabetic man presents with diabetic ketoacidosis. His systolic BP is 90 mmHg and his serum potassium is 6.5 mM

Q63   Acute blood loss of 2 litres in a previously healthy adult

Theme 2: Thyroid Cancer

A. Anaplastic carcinoma
B. Lymphoma

C. Follicular carcinoma
D. Medullary thyroid carcinoma
E. Papillary carcinoma
F. Thyroid sarcoma

For each of the patients described below, select the most likely diagnosis from the list of options above. Each option may be used once, more than once, or not at all.

Q64 A 26-year-old woman presents with a thyroid swelling. She is known to have Cushing's syndrome. Clinical examination demonstrates a 3 cm solid mass in the left thyroid lobe and hypertension (BP160/100 mm/Hg). Ultrasonography confirms the solid nature of the thyroid mass and FNAC showed malignant cells

Q65 A 17-year-old girl presents with a thyroid swelling. Clinical examination reveals a 2.5 cm solid mass in the right thyroid lobe and three enlarged cervical lymph nodes. Ultrasonography confirms the clinical findings. FNAC shows malignant cells with vesicular nuclei

Theme 3: Gastrointestinal Haemorrhage

A. Upper gastrointestinal (GI) endoscopy
B. Red blood cell scan
C. Colonoscopy
D. Selective angiography
E. Double contrast barium enema
F. Barium meal and follow through

For each of the patients described below, select the most likely investigation from the list of options above. Each option may be used once, more than once, or not at all.

Q66 A 50-year-old man presents to the Accident and Emergency Department with dizziness and melaena

Q67 A 65-year-old woman presents with dark red rectal bleeding, hypotension (BP 95/60 mm Hg), and tachycardia (pulse 100 bpm). FBC reveals anaemia (Hb 8.6 g/dl). Upper GI endoscopy shows no abnormality. Colonoscopy reveals dark red blood in the colon and no other abnormality

Q68 An anxious 20-year-old man, who has a strong family history of colorectal cancer, presents with a positive faecal occult blood test

Theme 4: Cancer Treatment

A. Cytotoxic chemotherapy
B. External beam radiotherapy
C. Radiotherapy and chemotherapy
D. Surgical excision of primary tumour
E. Hormonal manipulation

For each of the patients described below, select the most appropriate treatment from the list of options above. Each option may be used once, more than once, or not at all.

Q69 A 40-year-old woman presents with inflammatory carcinoma of the breast

Q70 A 50-year-old man presents with anal carcinoma (squamous cell) measuring 5 cm in diameter

Q71 A 75-year-old man presents with hepatomegaly. Investigations reveal metastatic carcinoma of the prostate

Q72 A 65-year-old woman presents with malignant cutaneous melanoma of the left arm

Theme 5: Cancer Prognosis

A. 95%
B. 70%
C. 50%
D. 30%
E. 12%

For each of the tumours described below, select the most likely survival rate at five years from the list of options above. Each option may be used once, more than once, or not at all.

Q73 Stage I seminoma treated by radiotherapy

Q74 Papillary thyroid carcinoma measuring 2 cm in size treated by total thyroidectomy, radioactive iodine and thyroxine

Q75 Ductal carcinoma *in situ* measuring 3 cm treated by total mastectomy

Q76 Carcinoma of the sigmoid colon (Dukes B) treated by sigmoid colectomy

Q77 Stage II cutaneous melanoma

Q78 Caecal carcinoma staged C2

Theme 6: Multiple Trauma

A. Haemothorax
B. Cardiac tamponade
C. Ruptured spleen
D. Flail chest
E. Tension pneumothorax
F. Aortic rupture

For each of the patients described below, select the most likely *single* diagnosis from the list of options above. Each option may be used once, more than once, or not at all.

Q79 A 24-year-old man is brought into the Accident and Emergency Department following a road traffic accident. He is conscious. He has tachypnoea (40 rpm), tachycardia (130 bpm) and distended neck veins. His systemic BP is 85/40 mmHg. His heart sounds are greatly diminished. A chest radiograph shows three fractured ribs (ribs 5, 6 and 7) on the left side and a small pneumothorax. A left chest drain and central venous catheter are inserted. The CVP is 20 cm. The BP is 90/50 mmHg after 2 litres of colloids infusion. The ECG shows reduced voltage in QRS complexes

Q80 A 50-year-old woman is brought into the Accident and Emergency Department following a road traffic accident. She is conscious with adequate airway. The GCS is 15. She is tachypnoeic (30 rpm). Her pulse is 150 bpm and reduced in volume. The distal pulses are present. Her BP is 85/45 mmHg. The chest radiograph shows multiple rib fractures on the left side (ribs 7, 8 and 9) and a 20% pneumothorax. A left chest drain is inserted (100 ml of blood is drained). The CVP is –2 cm. Analysis of the diagnostic peritoneal lavage (DPL) fluid reveals a WCC of 1000/mm^3 and an amylase level of 400 units. She remains hypotensive (BP 90/55 mmHg) despite the infusion of 5 units of colloids and 4 units of blood

Theme 7: The Acute Abdomen

A. Acute cholecystitis
B. Perforated peptic ulcer
C. Acute embolic mesenteric ischaemia
D. Small bowel obstruction
E. Acute pancreatitis
F. Acute diverticulitis

For each of the patients described below, select the most likely *single* diagnosis from the list of options above. Each option may be used once, more than once, or not at all.

Q81 A 62-year-old woman with a long-standing history of atrial fibrillation presents to the Accident and Emergency Department with a history of sudden onset of severe abdominal pain. She has had a large bowel movement since the onset of pain and vomited once. No flatus has been passed since that time. Clinical examination reveals a mildly distended abdomen which is diffusely tender. She has tachycardia (120 bpm), Kussmaul breathing and hypotension (100/50 mmHg). Her Hb is 13 g/dl, WCC is 23,000/mm^3, serum amylase 500 units, serum potassium 5.8 mmol/l and creatinine 160 µmol/l. Abdominal and chest radiographs have no diagnostic features. Ten years ago she underwent an abdominal hysterectomy

Q82 A 52-year-old man presents to the Accident and Emergency Department with a two-day history of severe epigastric pain of gradual onset radiating to the back and associated with nausea and vomiting. Clinical examination reveals tachycardia (120 bpm), tachypnoea (38 rpm), hypotension 95/60 mmHg), a tender mass in the upper abdomen and a periumbilical ecchymosis

Theme 8: Medicine and The Law

A. Any qualified doctor
B. Registrar of births and deaths
C. Coroner
D. Medical practitioner who attended the patient during previous 14 days
E. Expert witness

From the list above, select the most appropriate person to:

Q83 Issue an immediate death certificate

Q84 Certify death

Q85 Call an inquest

Q86 Send information regarding the cause of death to the office of Population Consensus and Survey (PCS)

Theme 9: Haematuria

A. Urinary tract infection (UTI)
B. Transitional cell carcinoma of the ureter
C. Renal adeno carcinoma
D. Ureteric calculus
E. Prostatic carcinoma
F. Prostatic hyperplasia

For each of the clinical presentations listed below, select the most appropriate diagnosis from the list of options above. Each option may be used once, more than once or not at all.

Q87   A 51-year-old man presents with a two-month history of haematuria and pain in the right flank. Urine microscopy confirms haematuria. (Hb = 19g/dl, WCC = 13 000/mm^3, haematocrit = 59%.)

Q88   A 20-year-old woman presents with urinary frequency, haematuria, and lower abdominal pain

Q89   A 75-year-old man presents with haematuria and backache. Plain radiographs show sclerotic areas in the lumbosacral spine

Q90   A 46-year-old worker in the rubber industry presents with haematuria and renal colic. A plain abdominal radiograph show no abnormality

Q91   A 35-year-old surgeon presents with severe flank pain, nausea and vomiting. Urine microscopy shows red blood cells and crystals. (Hb = 14g/dl and WCC = 15 000.)

Theme 10: Visual Field Defects

A. Bitemporal hemianopia
B. Contralateral homonymous hemianopia
C. Ipsilateral Homonymous hemianopia
D. Upper homonymous quadrantanopia
E. Lower homonymous quadrantanopia
F. Ipsilateral mononuclear field loss
G. Anton's syndrome

For the brain lesions described below, select the most appropriate resulting visual field defect from the list of options given above. Each option may be used once, more than once or not at all.

Q92   Optic nerve injury

Q93   Optic chiasmal injury

Q94   Parietal lobe injury

Q95   Temporal lobe injury

Q96   Unilateral occipital lobe injury

Q97   Optic tract injury

Q98   Bilateral occipital lobe injury

Answers

A1: A(T) B(T) C(T) D(T) E(F)
Intracellular components are released into the plasma from damaged cells, e.g. potassium, myoglobin, hydrogen ions, etc. Curling's ulcer is an example of stress ulceration which may occur in such patients. Metabolic acidosis is a recognised feature due to tissue hypoxia and cellular damage.

A2: A(T) B(T) C(F) D(F) E(T)
Level I axillary nodes lie lateral to the lateral border of the pectoralis minor muscle. Level II nodes lie behind the muscle and Level III nodes lie medial to the medial border of the P. minor muscle which is inserted into the coracoid process. The long thoracic nerve supplies the serratus anterior muscle and injury to the nerve leads to winging of scapula.

A3: A(F) B(F) C(T) D(F) E(T)
The reticular vessels travelling in the posterior capsule and the medullary vessels in the femoral neck proved most of the blood supply to the femoral head. The obturator branch reaches the head along the teres ligament and provides only 15% of the total blood supply to the femoral head. This minor supply is insufficient to maintain the viability of the femoral head if the other sources are damaged e.g. displaced subcapital fractures.

A4: A(T) B(F) C(T) D(T) E(T)
Figure 4 illustrates the tributaries of the long saphenous vein in the femoral triangle.

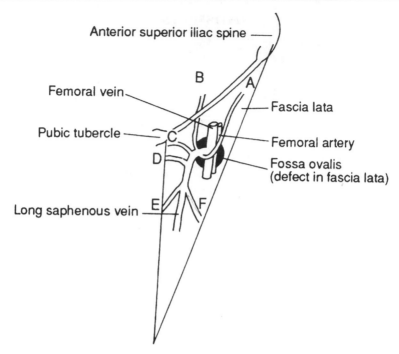

Figure 4   Femoral triangle showing entrance of the long saphenous vein through the fossa ovalis into the femoral vein. Tributaries of the long saphenous vein: A = superficial circumflex iliac; B = superficial epigastric; C = superficial external pudendal; D = deep external pudendal; E = medial femoral; F = lateral femoral.

A5: A(T)   B(F)   C(T)   D(T)   E(T)

Loss of axonal continuity is known as axonotmesis (e.g. crushing injury) whereas loss of nerve continuity (e.g. nerve section) is known as neurotmesis. Primary nerve repair is desirable in clean wounds, whereas delayed repair is preferable in the presence of contamination (3 to 4 weeks after injury).

A6: A(T)   B(T)   C(F)   D(T)   E(T)   F(F)

The internal diameter of the CBD is 6 mm on ultrasonography and 8 mm on cholangiography. CBD injury is more likely with laparo-scopic cholecystectomy, but the incidence decreases with increasing experience. The normally functioning gall bladder appears as a hot spot on the HIDA scan.

A7: A(F)   B(T)   C(T)   D(T)   E(F)

See Figure 5.

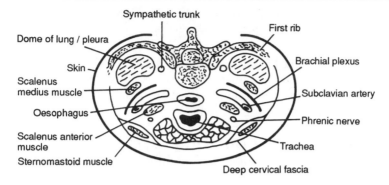

Figure 5   A transverse section through the root of the neck

A8: A(T)   B(F)   C(T)   D(F)   E(T)

The pH of the uniting fracture starts increasing after the tenth day (alkaline tide). Although hyperparathyroidism causes bore demineralisation, bore cysts and pathological fractures, there is no evidence that it impairs the process of fracture healing.

A9: A(F)   B(F)   C(T)   D(T)   E(T)   F(T)

Obstructive jaundices impairs the absorption of fat (steatorrhoea) and fat soluble vitamins such as vitamin K. The latter is important for the synthesis of clotting factors: II, VII, IX and X.

A10: A(F)   B(F)   C(F)   D(T)   E(T)

Crypt abscess are more conspicuous in ulcerative colitis (UC) and pseudopolyps are a striking feature of the disease. The risk of carcinoma complicating UC increases with time (approximately 15% at 20 years). Crohn's disease is characterised by granulomata and transural inflammation and is more likely to present with bowel obstruction

A11: A(F)   B(F)   C(T)   D(F)   E(T)

DCIS usually presents as screen-detected microcalcifications. It is characterised by malignant proliferation of ductal cells confined within the basement membrane. The incidence of lymph node metastasis is less than 1%. The comedo variety is high grade and is associated with a worse outcome. Approximately 65% of DCIS lesions develop into invasive cancer if left untreated for 10 years

A12: A(T)   B(T)   C(F)   D(T)   E(F)

In strenuous exercise, there is increased anaerobic metabolism leading to increased serum lactate and reduced pH. Heart rate, stroke volume and blood pressure rise. Damaged muscle fibres may lead to a rise in serum CPK.

A13: A(T) B(F) C(T) D(F) E(F) F(T)

Cholinergic stimulation causes detrusor muscle and gall bladder contraction. It also causes penile erection. Ejaculation is a function of the sympathetic nervous system.

A14: A(T) B(T) C(F) D(F) E(T)

Increased gastric acidity and secretin inhibit gastrin secretion.

A15: A(F) B(F) C(T) D(T) E(T) F(F)

Opening of the aortic valve coincides with the R-wave and closure occurs just after the T-wave, therefore during the P-wave the mitral valve is open and the aortic valve is closed. The first heart sound occurs at the beginning of the QRS complex whereas the second heart sound occurs just after the T-wave. The ECG features of hypokalaemia include prolonged QT segment, ST depression and T-wave inversion.

A16: A(F) B(T) C(T) D(F) E(F)

Hypoventilation increases PCO_2 and ICP. Mannitol is an osmotic diuretic that reduces CSF volume. Atracurium is a neuromuscular blocker that relaxes muscles and hence reduces intrathoracic pressure and ICP.

A17: A(T) B(F) C(T) D(T) E(F) F(F)

There is no evidence to support the widely-held belief that mild anaemia impairs wound healing. Corticosteroids inhibit epithelial-isation and fibroblast proliferation in healing wounds. Ultraviolet light promotes wound healing whereas hypoproteinaemia impairs the process. There is no evidence that jaundice per se impairs wound healing.

A18: A(F) B(F) C(T) D(F) E(T) F(F) G(F)

Primary hyperparathyroidism is most common in women aged 45–60 years. The condition is due to a parathyroid adenoma in most cases. The adenoma can be localised by a preoperative radioactive scan (Sestamibi scan). It is characterised by elevated serum calcium, and parathyroid hormone and decreased serum phosphate. The bone changes include demineralisation, bone cyst formation, osteo-blastomas and pathological fractures. However, fracture healing is not impaired. The condition affects the renal tract in more than

50% of cases and renal damage may lead to hypertension. Primary hyperparathyroidism is usually treated surgically by removal of the adenoma or hyperplastic glands.

A19: A(F) B(F) C(F) D(T) E(T)
Anaplastic tumours and those with short latency are not suitable for screening as early detection does not significantly improve outcome. Screening tests should be highly sensitive in order to minimise false negatives. Specificity is important for diagnostic tests which proceed definitive treatment. For example in breast cancer screening mammography has an acceptable sensitivity (approximately 85%), but we do not perform definitive breast cancer surgery on the basis of mammography only or the specificity is also approximately 85%. FNAC, however, has a specificity which exceeds 95% and can therefore be relied upon when planning treatment.

A20: A(T) B(T) C(T) D(F) E(T)
The diseased liver removes less antigens from the portal circulation resulting in hypergammaglobuminaemia. The liver synthesises most clotting factors, however factor VIII is synthesised by the vascular endothelium.

A21: A(T) B(F) C(F) D(T) E(F)
Fat embolus may arise from lipids in bone marrow and usually occurs within 24 hours of major fractures. It may cause confusion, hypoxia and haemorrhages in the dermis serum lipase is raised in a small proportion of causes. Pyoderma gangrenosum is a feature of inflammatory bowel disease.

A22: A(F) B(T) C(F) D(F) E(T)
In pseudohypoparathyroidism, there is failure of target cell response to PTH. The latter may be normal or raised. The physical signs include short metacarpals and metatarsals and round face. In acute pancreatitis some serum calcium binds to fatty acids liberated by lipase and the serum PTH is also reduced by the disease process. In sarcoidosis, there is increased 1-hydroxylation of 25-hydroxycholecalciferol by macrophages causing hypercalcaemia. The milk-alkali syndrome is another uncommon cause of hypercalcaemia.

A23: A(T) B(T) C(F) D(T) E(F)
Thiazide diuretics decrease urinary excretion of calcium whereas loop diuretics such as frusemide increase urinary excretion of

calcium. Bisphosphonates are used in the treatment of hyper-calcaemia and bony metastases. Pseudopsuedo hypoparathyroidism but the biochemistry is normal.

A24: A(T) B(T) C(F) D(T) E(F)
Cranial diabetes insipidus and hyperglycaemia cause polyuria. Conditions associated with excessive ADH secretion are associated with failure to excrete a waterload.

A25: A(F) B(T) C(F) D(F) E(T)
Hyperacute rejection is antibody mediated (cf. acute rejection which is cell-mediated). It is due to preformed antibodies caused by previous blood transfusions, pregnancy and/or previous failed transplants. It is treated by removal of transplant. Corticosteroids have a role in the treatment of acute rejection.

A26: A(F) B(T) C(T) D(F) E(F)
The incidence of hip dislocation is approximately 2%. Most disloca-tions occur within six months of surgery and are treated conserv-atively. Sciatic nerve injury complicates 1% of cases. Prophylactic antibiotics, gentamicin-impregnated cement and ultra-clean air en-closures have reduced infection rate. Loosening may be due to absorption of cement around the implant, hypersensitivity, low grade infection and/or imperfect prosthetic design.

A27: A(F) B(T) C(F) D(T) E(T)
Post-phlebotic syndrome occurs in 10% of patients with DVT. It presents with leg oedema, pain, nocturnal cramping, venous claudication, skin pigmentation, dermatitis and ulceration (usually on the medial aspect of the lower leg). In phlegmasia alba dolens, the leg is pale and cool with a diminished arterial pulse due to spasm. It usually results from acute occlusion of the iliac and femoral veins due to a DVT. In phlegmasia cerula dolens, there is an acute and nearly total venous occlusion of the entire extremity outflow, including the iliac and femoral veins. The leg is usually painful, cyanosed and oedematous. Venous gangrene may supervene. Milroy's disease is a congenital and inherited form of lymphoedema. Cystic hygromas are benign tumours derived from embryonic lymph sacs.

A28: A(F) B(T) C(F) D(T) E(F)
Nerves can survive ischaemia for 2–4 hours but can potentially regenerate. Muscle ischaemia may cause Volkmann's ischaemic

contractures. The forearm and lower leg compartments are the commonest sites. The presence of distal pulses does not exclude the syndrome. Extensive fasciotomy may be limb-saving.

A29: A(T) B(T) C(T) D(T) E(T)
Other complications include pneumothorax, dislodgement of the tube (partial or complete), obstruction of the tube or trachea, tracheal stenosis, sepsis, cuff prolapse, intubation granuloma of vocal cords. Subglottic stenosis occurs if the first and second tracheal rings are damaged.

A30: A(T) B(F) C(T) D(F) E(T) F(T)
The APC gene is located on the long arm of the chromosome 5. The syndrome presents in early adult life with rectal bleeding, abdominal pain and/or diarrhoea. More than 95% of patients develop colorectal carcinoma by the age of 40 years if the condition is left untreated. First degree relatives should be screened and treated (if affected) with colectomy and ileorectal anastomosis or proctocolectomy with a terminal ileostomy. If the rectum is preserved, it should be regularly screened with rigid sigmoidoscopy.

A31: A(F) B(T) C(F) D(F) E(F)
Male sex, increased tumour thickness, the presence of ulceration, older age and mucosal involvement are poor prognostic indicators. The prognosis also depends upon the lymph node involvement and growth pattern. The five-year survival rate is 90% for stage 1, 50% for stage II, 30% for stage III and < 1% for stage IV disease.

A32: A(T) B(F) C(F) D(T) E(F) F(T)
Cyclophosphamide is an alkylating agent which is activated by microsomal enzymes of the liver. Cyclophosphamide metabolites can cause haemorrhagic cystitis which can be prevented by maintaining a high urine flow and the administration of MESNA. Ifosfamide, which is equally effective is less myelotoxic.
Cyclophosphamide is used in the treatment of cancers of the ovary, breast, lung and testis. It is also used to treat sarcomas and lymphomas. The adverse effects include alopecia, nausea, vomiting, cardiotoxicity, testicular damage, myelotoxicity and carcinogenicity.

A33: A(F) B(T) C(T) D(F) E(F) F(T)
Gardner's syndrome is characterised by colorectal polyposis. It is transmitted by an autosomal dominant gene. The risk factors also include adenomatous polyposis coli, Lynch syndrome, ulcerative

colitis, low intake of dietary fibre, tobacco smoking, high intake of alcohol and dietary fat, family history of colorectal cancer and ureterosigmoidostomy.

A34: A(F) B(F) C(T) D(T) E(F) F(T)

The incidence of colorectal carcinoma is higher in developed countries than third world countries. This difference is thought to be due to a higher intake of fibre and a lower intake of red meat and animal fats in third world countries. Recent studies have suggested that FOB testing is an effective method of population screening. Serum carcinoembryonic antigen is the tumour marker for colorectal carcinoma. Right-sided lesions tend to present with microcytic anaemia. The fluid nature of the faeces and the lower incidence of stenosing lesions in the right colon explain the difference in clinical presentation between right and left colonic cancers. The latter tends to present with rectal bleeding and bowel obstruction. 5-Fluorouracil is the main chemotherapeutic agent used in the treatment of this disease.

A35: A(T) B(T) C(F) D(T) E(F) F(F) G(T)

Osteogenic sarcoma has two peaks of incidence: 10–25 years and 40–60 years. The common sites include the metaphysis of the femur (52%), proximal end of tibia (20%) and the humerus (9%). The male to female ratio is 3:2. 1% of patients suffering form Paget's disease of bone develop sarcoma. The tumour tends to spread towards the medulla and towards the periosteum. Involvement of the periosteum causes Codman's triangle on plain x-rays. The clinical features include pain, local tenderness, soft tissue mass and pathological bone fractures. The lung is a common site for metastatic disease. Pulmonary metastases can be resected with a five-year survival rate of 30%. The mainstay of management is adequate surgical excision and chemotherapy. Limb sparing surgery is possible in 80% of cases.

A36: A(F) B(F) C(T) D(T) E(F) F(T)

The right colic artery which may arise from the SMA or the ileocolic artery supplies the ascending colon and the hepatic flexure. The middle colic artery, a branch of the SMA, supplies the transverse colon. The left colic artery, a branch of the IMA, supplies the splenic flexure and the descending colon. The superior rectal artery arises from the IMA. The middle rectal artery arises from the internal iliac artery whereas the inferior rectal artery originates from the internal pudendal artery. The marginal artery connects the IMA (sigmoid and left colic branches) to the SMA (middle and right colic branches). The portosystemic anastomosis predisposes the haemorrhoids. The lymphatic drainage follows the blood supply.

A37: A(T) B(F) C(F) D(F) E(T) F(F) G(T)
Gastrointestinal lymphoma represents 5% of all gastrointestinal malignancies. The peak incidence occurs during the sixth and seventh decades. There are three main types:

1. Western lymphoma (non-Hodgkin's B-cell lymphoma)
2. Primary lymphoma associated with Coeliac disease (T-cell lymphoma), and
3. Mediterranean lymphoma associated with alpha chain disease

The clinical features include anaemia, abdominal pain, abdominal mass and symptoms and signs of obstruction, perforation or haemorrhage. Stage I and stage II disease are treated by surgical resection. Radiotherapy is indicated for high grade disease and positive margins. Stage III and IV disease are treated primarily by chemotherapy and radiotherapy. Surgery is reserved for complications in such cases.

A38: A(T) B(T) C(T) D(F) E(F) F(T) G(F) H(F)
Barrett's oesophagus is associated with a risk of 13% and requires regular endoscopic surveillance. Other risk factors include corrosive structures, Plummer–Vinson syndrome, tobacco smoking, alcohol and vitamin C deficiency. *Helicobacter pylori* is associated with gastric cancer. Alpha chain disease is a recognised risk factor for Mediterranean lymphoma.

A39: A(F) B(T) C(T) D(T) E(T) F(F) G(T)
Raised ICP leads to systemic hypertension and bradycardia (Cushing's reflex). Increased ICP may cause headaches, vomiting, papilloedema and tentorial herniation (with haemorrhage into the midbrain and pons). Battle's sign refers to bruising behind the ear and indicates a basal skull fracture.

A40: A(T) B(F) C(T) D(F) E(T)
Surgical drainage and thorough irrigation is the mainstay of management of this subcutaneous infection. I.V. antibiotics are also given guided by microbiological culture and sensitivity results. Inadequate treatment leads to adhesions and loss of function.

A41: A(T) B(T) C(T) D(F) E(F)

Many of the systemic complications of acute pancreatitis are mediated by cytokines such as IL-1 and TNF-α. Other complications include DIC, shock, hypoalbuminaemia, hypocalcaemia and acute tubular necrosis.

A42: A(F) B(T) C(F) D(T) E(F)

The external oblique fibres run parallel to the skin incision and Scarpa's fascia lies superficial to the external oblique muscle. The appendicular artery has no anastomoses and therefore the appendix is vulnerable to necrosis and perforation once the artery is occluded such as in inflammation.

A43: A(F) B(T) C(F) D(F) E(T)

The long saphenous vein (LSV) passes in front of the medial malleolus and usually lies anterior to the superficial external pudendal artery. The LSV has at least five tributaries near its junction with the deep femoral vein and this feature helps to distinguish the LSV from the deep femoral vein.

A44: A(F) B(F) C(T) D(F) E(T)

The latissimus dorsi muscle is supplied by the thoracodorsal artery and this myocutaneous flap is frequently used (as a pedicled flap) for breast reconstruction following mastectomy. The transverse rectus abdominis myocutaneous flap (TRAM) is supplied by the superior and inferior (deep) epigastric arteries. This myocutaneous flap is used for breast reconstruction as a free or pedided flap. The gracilis MF is supplied by the medial femoral circumflex artery.

A45: A(F) B(T) C(T) D(F) E(T)

The popliteal artery is the deepest structure in the popliteal fossa and lies lateral to the semitendinosus tendon. The artery is usually exposed through a medical approach when performing a femoro-popliteal bypass.

A46: A(F) B(T) C(T) D(T) E(F) F(F)

Most renal injuries are caused by blunt trauma and usually settle down with conservative management which includes regular observations and analgesia. CT is fairly accurate in the assessment of solid organ injuries. Angiography is considered if the traumatised kidney is not visible on IVU as this may suggest vascular avulsion. The long term complications of renal injuries include hypertension.

A47: A(T) B(T) C(F) D(F) E(F)
The relative contraindications also include morbid obesity and previous laparatomies. The positivity criteria for DPL include: WCC > 500 mm^{-3}, RBC > 100 000 mm^{-3}, fluid amylase > 200 units and the presence of gastrointestinal contents. DPL is more sensitive than CT scanning and false positives are rare.

A48: A(F) B(T) C(T) D(T) E(F)
The indications for thoracotomy following thoracic trauma include an initial drainage (haemothorax) greater than 1000 ml, cardiac tamponade and cardiorespiratory arrest. However, most thoracic injuries are managed by the insertion of a thoracostomy tube. Flail chest is usually managed conservatively with ventilation, analgesia and physiotherapy.

A49: A(F) B(T) C(F) D(F) E(T)
Significant blood loss leads to an increase in the rate of oxygen extraction (the haemoglobin – oxygen dissociation curve is shifted to the right), renin secretion and total peripheral resistance (vaso-constriction). Renin converts angiotensinogen into angiotensin I and the latter is converted by ACE in the lungs into angiotensin II. Angiotensin II stimulates aldosterone secretion (water and sodium retention) and causes vasoconstriction.

A50: A(T) B(F) C(F) D(F) E(F)
In court, expert witnesses should remember that they have a primary responsibility toward the judge. They are not immune to suing by clients.
Regarding negligence, the expert witness is usually experienced and specialist in the medical field in which the case arose but regarding causation this is not necessary.

A51: A(T) B(F) C(F) D(T) E(F)
The posterior column of the spinal cord transmits two-point discrimination, joint position and vibration sensory modalities.

A52: A(F) B(T) C(T) D(T) E(F) F(F) G(F)
The platysma, facial artery and vein and cervical branch of facial nerve lie superficial to the gland. The hypoglossal and lingual nerves and digastric muscle lie deep to the gland.

A53: A(F) B(T) C(T) D(F) E(T)
The brain receives 15% of total cardiac output (approximately

750 ml/min in a 70 kg healthy adult). The relationship between intracranial volume and pressure is not linear (Figure 6):

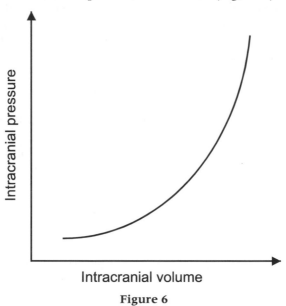

Figure 6

A54: A(F) B(T) C(T) D(F) E(T)
The atlanto-odontoid gap is 2.5 mm in adults and 4 mm in children. Swimmers view allows the assessment of the lower cervical vertebrae.

A55: A(T) B(T) C(F) D(F) E(T)
Cerebral blood flow is mainly controlled by the process of auto-regulation. Cerebral blood flow is increased by hypoxia and hypercapnia and automatic mechanisms seem to be unimportant.

A56: A(T) B(T) C(T) D(F) E(T) F(F)
Lumbar puncture is absolutely contraindicated in patients with intracranial mass lesions as the procedure could precipitate coning and death. Hyperventilation reduces PCO_2 and this reduces intra-cranial pressure (ICP) and is therefore desirable. Mannitol (1 g/kg as an i.v. 20% solution) is an osmotic diuretic that can reduce ICP.

A57: A(F) B(T) C(T) D(T) D(F)
Pericardial tamponade make the heart sound muffled and raises JVP. The combination of hypotension, muffled heart sounds and raised JVP is known as Beck's triad. The condition can be accurately diagnosed with echocardiography (two dimensional) and requires

surgical treatment (left anterior thoracotomy or medial sternotomy). Percutaneous needle aspiration may also help to establish the diagnosis.

A58: A(T) B(T) C(F) D(F) E(T) F(F) G(T)

The clinical signs of spinal cord injury include hypotension with relative bradycardia due to interruption of sympathetic outflow. Spinothalamic tract injury impairs contralateral pain and temperature sensations. Damage to the dorsal column impairs position, vibration (sensory ataxia) and two-point discrimination sensory modalities below the level of the lesion. The combination of spinothalamic and lateral corticospinal (ipsilateral pyramidal signs) tract injuries is known as Brown-Séquard syndrome.

A59: A(T) B(F) C(F) D(F) E(F)

The neck should be immobilised in all trauma patients and cervical spine injury should be considered in all cases. Adequate cervical spine X-rays are essential prior to excluding an injury especially in the unconscious patient. Conscious patients can be asked about pain in the cervical region and the spine can be reliably examined clinically, in such cases cervical spine X-rays are not required in every patient.

Experienced anaesthetists can intubate head injury patients without visualising the vocal cord.

Pressure on the cricoid cartilage during the intubation procedure is desirable in order to reduce the risk of aspiration. The passage of a nasogastric tube is contraindicated in patients with basal skull fractures.

A60: A(F) B(T) C(F) D(F) E(F)

Water accelerates the absorption of phenol and should be avoided in such burns. Intravenous fluids are required for burns > 15% in adults and > 10% in children. Routine use of antibiotics encourages the emergence of resistant organisms.

Haematocrit is usually maintained around 30% in critically ill patients.

A61: B

Haemaccel is isotonic with plasma and can be used to replace blood loss of up to one litre. Its half-life is approximately 6–8 hours.

A62: C

A63: E
Polygelatins are initially used then supplemented with blood (whole or packed cell) so that haematocrit is maintained around 30%.

A64: D
Medullary thyroid carcinoma is the only thyroid tumour associated with Cushing's syndrome. The hypertension may be due to Cushing's syndrome or an associated phaeochromocytoma. The most likely diagnosis in this patient is multiple endocrine neoplasia (MEN type IIa).

A65: E
The patient's age, the presence of cervical lymphadenopathy and the microscopic appearance of the nuclei makes papillary carcinoma the most likely diagnosis.

A66: A
Peptic ulceration is the commonest cause for such a presentation and therefore upper GI endoscopy is the investigation of choice in this patient. The procedure may also allow treatment, e.g. adrenline injection.

A67: B
RBC scan is a more sensitive investigation than selective angiography.

A68: C
Colonoscopy is a more accurate screening test than double contrast barium enema. However, the latter is cheaper and associated with lower morbidity and mortality rates. In view of the family history and positive FOB test, colorectal polyps should be excluded. Polyps smaller than 1 cm in size can be easily missed by barium enema.

A69: C
Inflammatory carcinoma is a totally advanced cancer by definition. Failure of response is an indication for mastectomy.

A70: C
SCC carcinoma of the anus is best treated by radiotherapy and chemotherapy (mitomycin C and 5-FU). Failure of response is an indication for surgical excision.

A71: E

A72: D
Surgical excision of the malignant skin lesion and sentinel node biopsy. If the latter is positive, then regional lymph node dissection is performed.

A73: A

A74: A

A75: A

A76: C

A77: D

A78: E

A79: B

A80: C
Hypotension, tachycardia and low CVP suggest hypovolaemia. Multiple rib fractures on the left-side and positive DPL support the diagnosis of splenic rupture.

A81: C
The sudden onset of the pain, atrial fibrillation and bowel opening support this diagnosis. The Kussmaul breathing and hyperkalaemia may be due to associated metabolic acidosis. Further investigations include arterial blood gas analysis and mesenteric angiography.

A82: E
The gradual onset of pain, the radiation to the back, the peri-umbilical ecchymosis (Cullen's sign) and the hypoxaemia make acute pancreatitis most likely.

A83: D

A84: A

A85: C

A86: B

A87: C
The presence of polycythaemia (raised Hb and raised haematocrit) favours the diagnosis of renal cell carcinoma.

A88: A
The patient's age and symptoms make UTI the most likely diagnosis.

A89: E
The backache and sclerotic lesions are consistent with prostatic carcinoma secondaries.

A90: B
Working in the rubber and aniline industries is a risk factor. The normal plain radiograph makes renal calculus less likely (90% of renal calculi are radio opaque).

A91: D
Being a surgeon is a risk factor for renal calculi (relative risk = 5). The presence of crystals in urine supports the diagnosis which can be confirmed by intravenous urography.

A92: F

A93: A

A94: E

A95: D

A96: B

A97: B

A98: G

System Modules Paper A

Questions

Q1   Acute appendicitis:

A. Has a peak incidence in the fourth decade
B. May cause microscopic haematuria
C. Usually presents with vomiting followed by abdominal pain
D. May cause diarrhoea
E. Complicated by an appendix mass, should be initially treated conservatively

Q2   Pancreatic pseudocysts:

A. Raise serum amylase
B. Are lined by epithelial tissue
C. Usually present with acute abdominal pain
D. May resolve spontaneously
E. Should be excised surgically

Q3   Aortic graft infection:

A. Is usually due to staphylococcus aureus
B. Is occasionally caused by helicobacter pylori
C. May occur 10 years after surgery
D. Responds to conservative treatment in almost all cases
E. Incidence is reduced significantly by using perioperative anti-microbials

Q4   Recognised complications of abdominal aortic aneurysm repair include:

A. Ischaemic colitis
B. Trash foot
C. Paraplegia
D. Incisional hernia
E. Madura foot

Q5   Ruptured abdominal aortic aneurysm (AAA):

A. Diagnosis should be confirmed by CT scanning prior to surgery
B. May raise serum amylase
C. Repair may be complicated by aorto-duodenal fistula
D. Is usually repaired with a woven Dacron graft
E. Has a mortality rate of 10%

Q6   Carcinoma of the parotid gland is:

A. The commonest malignant tumour of the salivary glands
B. A recognised complication of pleomorphic adenoma
C. A recognised cause of facial nerve palsy
D. A radio resistant tumour
E. Associated with a ten-year survival of 50% for high-grade tumours

Q7   Cancer of the lip:

A. Has a higher incidence among blacks
B. Is usually squamous cell carcinoma (SCC)
C. Usually occurs at the angle of the mouth
D. Tends to metastasise to submandibular nodes
E. Is radiosensitive

Q8   The following treatment modalities have been shown to prolong survival of patients with breast cancer:

A. Adjuvant tamoxifen in post menopausal patients
B. Adjuvant systemic chemotherapy
C. Removal of axillary nodes
D. Mastectomy compared with quadrantectomy
E. Bilateral salpingo oophorectomy in premenopausal patients
F. Post-operative radiotherapy in node-positive patients undergoing mastectomy

Q9   In the management of early breast cancer:

A. Axillary dissection prolongs survival
B. Mastectomy is associated with higher survival rates than conservative surgery
C. Post-operative radiotherapy reduces the incidence of local recurrence
D. Adjuvant tamoxifen has reduced mortality in post menopausal patients
E. Systemic chemotherapy has improved local control but not overall survival

Q10 **When investigating a breast lesion, fine needle aspiration cytology 'FNAC':**

A. Specificity exceeds 95%
B. Sensitivity exceeds 95%
C. Can be performed for impalpable breast lesions
D. Can distinguish between infiltrating and *in situ* breast lesions
E. Is more specific than core biopsy (Tru-cut)

Q11 **Renal calculi:**

A. Presents with macroscopic haematuria in most cases
B. Are radio opaque in most cases
C. Respond to conservative treatment in most cases
D. Complicated by pyelonephritis, should be treated with urgent extracorporeal shock wave lithotripsy (ESWL)
E. Are best investigated with intravenous urography

Q12 **The following are recognised medical treatments for benign prostatic hyperplasia (BPH):**

A. Prazosin
B. Finasteride
C. Oxybutynin
D. Goserelin
E. Alfuzosin

Q13 **Recognised causes of Raynaud's phenomenon include:**

A. Cryoglobulinaemia
B. Intra-arterial papavarine administration
C. Scleroderma
D. Macroglobulinaemia
E. Idiopathic thromboctyopenic purpura
F. Thoracic outlet syndrome
G. Phenoxybenzamine therapy

Q14 **Compared with synthetic vascular grafts, autogenous vein grafts are:**

A. Less thrombogenic
B. More difficult to revise
C. Less likely to be patent at 5 years

Q15   Abdominal aortic aneurysms (AAAs):

A. Are due to diabetes mellitus in most cases
B. Usually expand at 10 mm per year
C. May be caused by salmonella
D. Are inflammatory in 7% of cases
E. Measuring 7 cm in diameter, have a 5-year rupture rate of 40%

Q16   The following are recognised treatments for leg ulcers secondary to arterial insufficiency:

A. Compression stockings
B. Surgical debridement
C. Femoro popliteal bypass
D. Leg elevation
E. Ligation of the sapheno femoral junction

Q17   The following are recognised treatment modalities for epistaxis:

A. Compressing the nostrils between the finger and thumb for 10 minutes
B. Intranasal GTN spray
C. 5% cocaine spray combined with cauterisation
D. Foley catheter with the balloon lying in the anterior nasal space
E. Ligation of the anterior ethmoid artery via the orbit

Q18   Recognised complications of sclerotherapy for varicose veins include:

A. Trash foot
B. Brown discoloration of the skin
C. DVT
D. Ulceration of the skin
E. Sudeck's dystrophy

Q19   Benign prostatic hyperplasia (BPH):

A. Mainly affects the peripheral zone
B. Is a recognised cause of elevated serum PSA
C. Incidence is increased in males castrated before puberty
D. Symptoms improve with oxybutynin
E. Can be treated with 5-α-reductase inhibitors

Q20   Cystic hygromas:

A. Are the commonest benign tumours of the lymphatics
B. Occur most commonly in the groin
C. May occur in the mediastinum
D. Are commonly treated with radiotherapy
E. Should be excised completely even if cranial nerves are sacrificed

Q21   Recognised complications of percutaneous nephrolithotomy include:

A. Interstitial cystitis
B. Pyelovenous reflux of irrigating fluid
C. Ureteric obstruction
D. Haemorrhage
E. Arteriovenous fistula

Q22   The following are recognised surgical treatments for lymphoedema:

A. Homans' operation
B. Lymphovenous microanastomosis
C. Long saphenous vein transposition
D. Trendelenburg's operation
E. Mesenteric bridge operation

Q23   Thyroglossal cyst:

A. Results from embryological failure of the thyroglossal tract to obliterate
B. Usually presents during the middle age
C. Located in the subhyoid position in most cases
D. Contains lymphoid tissue
E. Is pre-malignant

Q24   In Trendelenburg's operation for varicose veins:

A. The patient is placed supine with $30°$ of head-up tilt
B. The sapheno-femoral junction (SFJ) lies 2 cm lateral and 2 cm below the pubic tubercle
C. The femoral vein has several tributaries near the SFJ
D. The long saphenous vein (LSV) is ligated and divided near the SFJ
E. A good outcome is expected if the LSV is a collateral for obstructed deep veins

Q25   Intertrochanteric fractures of the femur:

A. Cause shortening and external rotation of the lower limb
B. Usually cause the leg to become abducted
C. Significantly compromise the blood supply to the femoral head in most cases
D. Are best treated by hemiarthroplasty with femoral head replacement
E. Can be treated with dynamic hip screw (DHS) fixation

Q26   Salivary calculi:

A. Consist of calcium oxalate in most cases
B. Affect the parotid gland in most cases
C. Incidence is decreased by regular tooth brushing
D. Occasionally necessitate a complete excision of the involved gland
E. Commonly present with sialadenitis
F. May be treated by acidifying saliva

Q27   Primary hyperparathyroidism is:

A. Caused by hyperplasia in 50% of cases
B. A recognised cause of bone cysts
C. A recognised cause of constipation
D. A recognised complication of chronic renal failure
E. Characterised by hyperphosphataemia

Q28   Undescended testis:

A. Occurs in 7% of boys
B. Is more commonly seen on the right-side
C. Is usually hyperplastic
D. May be treated with LHRH agonists
E. Malignancy risk is eliminated with orchidopexy

Q29   In the management of renal stones, the contraindications to percutaneous nephrolithotomy (PCNL) include:

A. Abdominal aortic aneurysms
B. Stones in a transplanted kidney
C. Stones that cannot be positioned within the focus of the shock waves
D. Urinary obstruction not caused by the stone itself
E. Large volume stones

Q30   The following are recognised causes of priapism:

A. Leukaemia
B. Cycling
C. Sickle cell disease
D. Noradrenaline
E. Suxamethonium

Q31   In the management of Colles' fractures:

A. Anaesthesia can be achieved by injecting a local anaesthetic into the fracture haematoma
B. The wrist should be kept in extension following reduction
C. The hand should be in radial deviation after reduction
D. The plaster back slab should be completed immediately after adequate reduction
E. The plaster should extend above the elbow

Q32   Colles' fracture:

A. Is relatively common in women under the age of 50 years
B. Usually results from a fall on an outstretched hand
C. Causes 'dinner fork' deformity
D. Is reduced by applying traction, flexion and radial deviation
E. Is a recognised cause of Sudeck's atrophy

Q33   Risk factors for breast cancer include:

A. Smoking
B. Premenopausal obesity
C. Early menopause
D. Nulliparity
E. Atypical epithelial hyperplasia in a previous breast biopsy
F. Hormone replacement therapy

Q34   In the management of a simple (no tissue loss) contaminated wound of the upper limb which is seen 12 hours after injury:

A. 250 units of human tetanus immunoglobulin should be given if the patient is not actively immunised
B. Systemic benzylpenicillin is indicated
C. The wound should be closed immediately with non-absorbable sutures
D. The wound can be safely closed 5 days later after initial cleaning and regular dressings
E. Active tetanus immunisation is not indicated if passive immunisation is given

Q35   The causes of carpal tunnel syndrome include:

A. Thyrotoxicosis
B. Pregnancy
C. Cervical spondylitis
D. Cervical rib
E. Rheumatoid arthritis

Q36   Recognised complications of arteriovenous malformations (AVMs) include:

A. Cardiac failure
B. Haemorrhage
C. Unequal limb length
D. Madura foot
E. Dilated cardiomyopathy

Q37   In acute otitis media:

A. *Staphylococcus aureus* is the commonest causative bacterium
B. Perforation of the tympanic membrane is characterised by worsening the pain
C. Epileptic fits are a recognised complication
D. Ciprofloxacin is the antibiotic of choice
E. Myringotomy is a recognised treatment modality

Q38   Acute tonsillitis:

A. Is caused by viruses in approximately 50% of cases
B. Related rheumatic fever is prevented by use of antibiotics
C. Complicated by quinsy is an indication for tonsillectomy
D. Is a recognised cause of a retropharyngeal abscess
E. Is best treated by amoxycillin

Q39   The clinical features of maxillary sinusitis include:

A. Simple cheek swelling
B. Toothache
C. Purulent nasal discharge
D. Impaired sense of smell
E. Bell's palsy

Q40   With reference to conjunctivitis:

A. Most cases are unilateral
B. The intraocular pressure is normal
C. Adenoviruses are a recognised cause
D. Chloramphenicol ointment is the treatment of choice in chlamydial conjunctivitis
E. Sodium cromoglycate eye drops are effective in allergic cases

Q41   Following subtotal thyroidectomy:

A. Serum calcium should be estimated daily for at least 3 days after surgery
B. A pair of clip removing forceps should be available on the surgical ward where the patient is nursed
C. Stridor and cyanosis are pathognomonic of bilateral recurrent laryngeal nerve injury
D. Tetany is treated with i.v. calcium
E. Abducted vocal cords indicate recurrent laryngeal nerve injury

Q42   L-Thyroxine:

A. Is mainly absorbed in the duodenum
B. Half-time is approximately 2 days
C. Is more tightly bound to plasma proteins than T3
D. Has a quicker action than T3
E. Is available in an injectable form

Q43   In thyroid crisis, the following are recognised treatment:

A. Dexamethasone
B. Propylthiouracil
C. Plasmapheresis
D. Glucagon
E. Octreotide

Q44   In the management of parotid adenomas:

A. Enucleation has a similar local recurrence rate to wide local excision
B. Fine needle aspiration carries a risk of implantation recurrence
C. Post-operative radiation following enucleation reduced local recurrence rate to almost zero
D. Enucleation significantly reduces the incidence of facial nerve injury compared with wide local excision
E. An S-shaped cervicofacial incision is used for superficial parotidectomy

Q45   Wilms' tumour:

A. Is bilateral in about 10% of cases
B. Classically presents with haematuria as an early symptom
C. Is staged as IV if it is bilateral
D. Stage I is best treated with radiotherapy
E. Gene is located on chromosome 5

Q46   Recognised sites for ectopic testis include:

A. Perineum
B. Space of Burn's
C. Scarpa's triangle
D. True pelvis
E. Urethral diverticulum

Q47   Recognised treatment modalities for bleeding oesophageal varices include:

A. Beta blockers
B. Vasopressin
C. Phenol sclerotherapy
D. Splenorenal shunt
E. Omeprazole

Q48　Paraoesophageal hiatus hernia:

A. Accounts for 40% of all hiatus hernias
B. Usually presents before the age of 30 years
C. Is excluded in the presence of oesophagitis
D. Is a recognised indication for fundoplication
E. Is an indication for surgical repair once diagnosed

Q49　Colonic pseudo-obstruction:

A. Is also known as Ogilvie syndrome
B. Is a contraindication to a colonoscopy
C. May be treated with endoscopic caecostomy
D. Is painless in almost all cases
E. Diagnosis is often confirmed by a contrast enema
F. Is excluded if bowel sounds are present

Q50　Acute cholecystitis:

A. May occur in the absence of gallstones
B. Is a contraindication to laparoscopic cholecystectomy in the first 48 hours
C. Typically causes a 'hot spot' on the HIDA scan
D. Is a recognised cause of peritonitis
E. Complicated by empyema, can be treated by percutaneous drainage

Q51　Acute pancreatitis:

A. Is excluded if serum amylase is normal in a patient presenting with acute abdominal pain
B. Severity is accurately assessed with serial ultrasonography
C. Is an absolute contraindication to ERCP
D. Related mortality is reduced by the use of octreotide
E. Associated with the presence of three Ransom's criteria on admission, has a 10% mortality risk

Q52　Volvulus of the sigmoid colon:

A. Usually occurs in a clockwise direction
B. Is usually diagnosed on plain abdominal radiographs
C. Is initially treated by gentle untwisting with the rigid sigmoidoscopy
D. Associated with gangrene of the sigmoid colon, is treated by Hartmann's procedure
E. Has a recurrence rate of 90% with non-operative management

Q53   In the management of endoscopic perforation of the oesophagus:

A. Barium swallow is the investigation of choice
B. Conservative management is less likely to be successful than in spontaneous rupture cases
C. Conservative management is recommended for perforations less than 1 cm in size
D. Middle third perforations requiring surgery are approached through a right thoracotomy
E. Surgical repair is recommended for a perforation measuring 2.5 cm

Q54   Recognised complications of ulcerative colitis include:

A. Pyoderma gangrenosum
B. Primary biliary cirrhosis
C. Rectal carcinoma
D. Colonic perforation
E. Carcinoid tumours of the colon

Q55   Familial adenomatous polyposis (FAP):

A. Is transmitted in an autosomal dominant fashion
B. Gene is located on the short arm of chromosome 5
C. Is rarely complicated by carcinoma before the age of 39 years
D. May affect the small intestine
E. Is usually treated by total colectomy

Q56   Carcinoma of the pancreatic head:

A. Is associated with H-ras oncogene in most cases
B. Typically presents with obstructive jaundice and non-palpable gallbladder
C. Is highly radiosensitive
D. Causes a rise in serum CA19-9
E. Is accurately staged with trans-abdominal ultrasonography

Q57   In the management of haemorrhoids:

A. Sclerotherapy is the treatment of choice for third degree haemorrhoids
B. Prostatitis is a recognised complication of injection sclerotherapy
C. Injection sclerotherapy is effective in 90% of patients with first degree haemorrhoids
D. Haemorrhoidectomy may be complicated by anal stenosis
E. Anal dilatation under GA is the treatment of choice in frail, elderly subjects

Q58   Gallstones:

A. Made of pure cholesterol, are the commonest variety
B. Are a recognised cause of small bowel obstruction
C. Incidence is reduced in patients with inflammatory bowel disease
D. Can be diagnosed by ultrasonography with accuracy exceeding 90%
E. Can be treated with extracorporeal shock wave lithotripsy

Q59   Pancreatic pseudocyst:

A. Takes one week to mature
B. Is lined by an epithelial layer
C. Usually presents with acute abdominal pain
D. Can be treated by cystojejunostomy
E. May resolve spontaneously

Q60   In the management of gallstones:

A. Dissolution therapy with ursodeoxycholic acid is suitable for calcified gallstones in elderly patients
B. Dissolution therapy requires a functioning gallbladder
C. Extracorporeal shock wave lithotripsy (ESWL) is a recognised treatment modality for stones < 2 cm in size
D. Transduodenal sphincterotomy is indicated for a calculus impacted in the ampulla and cannot be extracted via ERCP
E. Choledochojejunostomy is strongly indicated for suppurative cholangitis complicating stones in the CBD

Theme 1: Renal Calculi

A. Percutaneous nephrolithotomy (PCNL)
B. Extracorporeal shock wave lithotripsy (ESWL)
C. Alkaline diuresis

D. Nephrectomy
E. Percutaneous nephrostomy
F. Expectant therapy

For each of the following cases listed below, select the most likely single treatment from the options listed above. Each option can be used once, more than once or not at all.

Q61 A 30-year-old pregnant woman (26 weeks) presents with septicaemia and abdominal pain. Investigations reveal an obstructed right kidney due to a 2 cm calculus. She is commenced on iv antimicrobials

Q62 A 40-year-old man presents with a left-side renal colic. IVU shows a 1 cm calculus in the upper third of his ureter. There is no complete obstruction. His symptoms fail to resolve on conservative management

Q63 A 20-year-old man presents with a renal colic secondary to a 1 cm cystine calculus

Q64 A 30-year-old man presents to the casualty department with a right-sided renal colic. An IVU shows a 4 mm calculus in the distal part of the ureter with no complete obstruction

Q65 A 40-year-old woman is found to have a staghorn calculus in a non-functioning kidney

Q66 A 60-year-old man presents with frequent attacks of left-side renal colic due to a 2.5 cm calculus in the renal pelvis. He has cardiac pacemaker and is known to have a 6 cm aortic aneurysm

Theme 2: Laryngeal Cancer

A. Total laryngectomy ± neck dissection
B. Radiotherapy
C. Chemotherapy
D. Hemilaryngectomy (vertical)
E. Supraglottic laryngectomy (horizontal) ± neck dissection
F. Excision of vocal cord mucosa

For each of the presentations below, select the most likely single treatment from the options listed above. Each option can be used once, more than once or not at all.

Q67 A 50-year-old man presents with a hoarse voice. Clinical examination and investigations reveal a small invasive carcinoma of the right vocal cord. The right vocal cord is paralysed and there is a 4 cm lymph node in the right anterior neck

Q68 A 65-year-old man is found to have a T1 carcinoma of the vocal cord. There is no involvement of the anterior commissure

Q69 A 60-year-old woman is found to have carcinoma *in situ* of the left vocal cord

Q70 A 55-year-old woman is found to have a glottic carcinoma involving the anterior commissure

Q71 A fit 70-year-old woman with large supraglottic carcinoma

Theme 3: Thyrotoxicosis

A. Radioactive iodine
B. Subtotal thyroidectomy
C. Propanalol
D. Carbimazole
E. Potassium iodide
F. Thyroxine

For each of the presentations below, select the most likely single treatment from the options listed above. Each option can be used once, more than once or not at all.

Q72 A 26-year-old pregnant woman is found to have thyrotoxicosis due to Grave's disease during the second trimester of the pregnancy

Q73 A 10-year-old girl presents with thyrotoxicosis. A radioactive radioisotope scan shows an enlarge thyroid with uniform uptake throughout

Q74 A 30-year-old woman is found to have Grave's disease. She remains thyrotoxic after treatment with carbimazole for 1 year

Q75 A 60-year-old woman is found to have a large toxic nodular goitre

Q76 A 50-year-old woman presents with a thyroid enlargement. Thyroid function tests are normal. The needle biopsy confirms the diagnosis of Hashimoto's thyroiditis

Theme 4: Pancreatic and Hepatobiliary Disease

A. Carcinoma of the head of the pancreas
B. Chronic pancreatitis
C. Primary biliary cirrhosis
D. Mirizzi's syndrome
E. Cholangiocarcinoma
F. A stone in the CBD

For each of the patients described below, select the most likely single diagnosis from the list above. Each option can be used once, more than once or not at all.

Q77 A 67-year-old man presents with a six month history of upper abdominal pain radiating to his back, associated with steatorrhoea and weight loss. Clinical examination reveals jaundice, a palpable left supraclavicular lymph node and a palpable gallbladder. Haematology and serum biochemistry reveals anaemia (Hb 10 g/dl) and deranged liver function tests (ALP 970 U/l, AST 270 U/l, ALT 275 U/l, bilirubin 89 µmol/l)

Q78 A 35-year-old woman presents with upper abdominal pain and nausea. Clinical examination reveals jaundice and no other abnormality. She had a laparoscopic cholecystectomy three weeks ago. Dipstick testing of urine demonstrates bilirubin. FBC is normal. Serum biochemistry shows abnormal liver function tests (bilirubin 75 µmol/litre, ALP 720 U/l, AST 170 U/l, GGT 100 U/l and ALT 190 U/l) and mildly raised amylase. The CBD diameter is 15 mm on ultrasonography, which shows no other abnormality

Theme 5: Hepatic Cancer

A. Hepatectomy
B. Radiotherapy
C. Chemotherapy
D. Tamoxifen
E. Liver transplantation

For each of the patients described below, select the most appropriate treatment from the list above. Each option can be used once, more than once or not at all.

Q79 A 70-year-old man presents with abdominal pain and hepato-megaly. Investigations reveal a multinodular hepatocellular carcinoma. He has a history of unstable angina and peripheral vascular disease

Q80 A 64-year-old woman presents with upper abdominal pain. Investigations show a 3 cm hepatoma arising in the left lobe. Her liver function tests are normal

Theme 6: Painful Swollen Knee

A. Osteoarthritis
B. Rheumatoid arthritis
C. Collateral ligament injury
D. Cruciate ligament injury
E. Patellar fracture
F. Tibial platau fracture

For each of the cases listed below, select the most appropriate diagnosis from the options listed above. Each option may be used once, more than once or not at all.

Q82 A 20-year-old man presents with a painful swollen knee after twisting his knee while in flexion in a football game. Needle aspiration reveals blood.

Q83 A 60-year-old woman presents with a painful swollen knee after a fall. She is unable to extend her knee. Aspiration shows blood and fat globules.

Theme 7: Jaundice

A. Primary biliary cirrhosis
B. Chronic active hepatitis
C. Carcinoma of the head of pancreas
D. Sclerosing cholangiatitis
E. Cholangiocarcinoma
F. Primary hepatocellular carcinoma
G. Gilbert's syndrome
H. Dubin-Johnson syndrome
I. Stones in common bile duct (CBD)

For each of the following clinical history, select the most likely diagnosis from the list of options above.

Q84 A 12-year-old boy presents with jaundice after a recent episode of tonsillitis. Serum bilirubin rises further on fasting. USS and liver biopsy reveal no abnormality.

Q85 A 27-year-old man presents with jaundice. He also describes a six month history of bloody diarrhoea. Hb is 10 g/dl, bilirubin is 75 µmol/l, AST/ALT/ALP/GGT are raised. LFT's improve with ursodeoxycholic acid administration.

Q86 A 45-year-old woman presents with painless jaundice 4 weeks after laparoscopic cholecystectomy, serum bilirubin = 105 µmol/l, AST = 150 U/L, ALP = 750 U/L.

Q87 A 69-year-old woman presents with jaundice and backache. Clinical examination shows a mass in the right upper quadrant, acanthosis nigricans and superficial thrombophlebitis.

Q88 A 49-year-old woman with Sjögren's syndrome presents with jaundice and hepatosplenomegaly. Her urine is dark and serum contains antimitochondrial antibody. (titres > 1:80), liver biopsy shows ductal destruction, proliferation and granulomata.

Answers

A1: A(F) B(T) C(F) D(T) E(T)
The peak incidence of acute appendicitis occurs during the second and third decades. It is rare at the extremes of age. The sequence of vomiting followed by abdominal pain should cast doubt over the diagnosis of acute appendicitis. Appendix mass is usually treated conservatively with antimicrobials and percutaneous drainage of pus if indicated. The presence of haematuria and diarrhoea should not exclude the diagnosis

A2: A(T) B(F) C(F) D(T) E(F)
Pancreatic pseudocysts consist of inflammatory products from neighbouring organs. They take 3–6 weeks to mature. Pancreatic pseudocysts usually present with low grade fever, leukocytosis, chronic abdominal pain and/or persistent rise in serum amylase. They are treated with percutaneous (with imaging guidance), internal or external drainage

A3: A(T) B(F) C(T) D(F) E(T)
H. pylori has not been reported as a cause of aortic graft infection. Surgical treatment (radical or limited) is often necessary

A4: A(T) B(T) C(T) D(T) E(F)
Paraplegia may result from injury to the artery of Adamkiewicz. Ligation of the inferior mesenteric artery in the absence adequate collateral circulation to the left colon may cause ischaemic colitis. Madura foot is infective in origin.

A5: A(F) B(T) C(T) D(T) E(F)
If the diagnosis is uncertain and the patient is stable, then CT scanning may have a role in establishing the diagnosis. The aneurysm wall is usually used to cover the synthetic graft. Avoidance of inadvertent injury to the duodenum and coverage of the synthetic graft help to reduce the incidence of aortoduodenal fistula. The mortality rate of ruptured AAA is ≥ 50%

A6: A(T) B(T) C(T) D(F) E(F)
The risk factors for carcinoma of the parotid gland include pleomorphic adenoma, and previous radiotherapy. The histological

grade is more predictive of prognosis and behaviour than the histological type. The diagnosis is usually confirmed by core biopsy (or FNAC). The mainstay of the treatment is surgical excision. Radiotherapy is indicated for high grade lesions. The 10 year survival rate is 90% for low grade tumours and 25% for high grade ones.

A7: A(F) B(T) C(F) D(T) E(T)

The incidence of lip cancer is higher among Caucasians, smokers and outdoor workers. SCC is the commonest histological type. Basal cell carcinoma is occasionally seen. 92% of lesions occur in the lower lip, 5% in the upper lip and 3% at the angle of mouth. Surgery and radiotherapy are equally effective.

A8: A(T) B(T) C(F) D(F) E(T) F(T)

Adjuvant systemic chemotherapy has reduced breast cancer mortality by 30%. The indications for systemic chemotherapy include positive axillary nodes, negative oestrogen receptors, poorly differentiated and large tumours in fit patients.

Axillary dissection provides important prognostic information and reduces the incidence of regional recurrence. No survival benefit has been demonstrated with radiotherapy which seems to reduce the local recurrence rate. Mastectomy is superior to conservative surgery in controlling local disease, but the addition of radiotherapy to conservative surgery results in similar local control rates.

A9: A(F) B(F) C(T) D(T) E(F)

The mainstay of management of early breast cancer consists of a wide local excision of the primary tumour combined with removal of the axillary nodes and followed by radiotherapy. Such management has similar survival and local control rates to mastectomy. Axillary dissection provides valuable prognostic information and improves loco regional control Adjuvant systemic therapy has reduced mortality by 30%.

A10: A(T) B(F) C(T) D(F) E(F)

The specificity of FNAC exceeds 98% in the hands of experienced cytologists. However, a negative result does not exclude the diagnosis of malignancy. FNAC can be performed stereotactically for impalpable lesions but it is not possible to distinguish between invasive and *in situ* tumours.

Core biopsy allows a formal histological diagnosis and is more specific (almost 100%) than FNAC.

A11: A(F) B(T) C(T) D(F) E(T)
Renal calculi are radiopaque in 90% of cases. IVU is the invest-igation of choice. If the calculus is causing complete obstruction and pyelonephritis, then urgent drainage with percutaneous neph-rostomy (under ultrasound guidance) is required in order to save the kidney. Sepsis is a contraindication to ESWL. Renal calculi up to 5 mm in size can be managed conservatively. Larger calculi often require ESWL, percutaneous, open or endoscopic extraction.

Macroscopic haematuria is occasionally seen, whereas micro-scopic haematuria is seen in most cases.

A12: A(T) B(T) C(F) D(F) E(T)
Prazosin and alfuzosin are selective alpha blockers which relax prostatic smooth muscles. Finasteride is a specific inhibitor of 5-alpha reductase which metabolises testosterone into the more potent androgen dihydrotestosterone. It is an effective alternative to alpha blockers especially in larger prostates.

Oxybutynin is an anti-muscarinic drug which is used in the treatment of urinary frequency due to bladder instability.

Goserelin is an LHRH-analogue which has a role in the treatment of prostatic cancer.

A13: A(T) B(F) C(T) D(T) E(F) F(T) G(F)
Scleroderma is the most commonly associated condition. Papavarine and phenoxybenzamine cause arterial vasodilatation. Thrombocytosis and not ITP is associated with Raynaud's phenomenon.

A14: A(T) B(T) C(F)
The 5-year patency rate is higher for autogenous vein grafts.

A15: A(F) B(F) C(T) D(T) E(F)
AAs are caused by atherosclerosis in most cases. They expand at approximately 4 mm per year. Mycotic aneurysms may be caused by salmonella. The 5-year rupture rate for aneurysms measuring 7 cm is approximately 75%.

A16: A(F) B(T) C(T) D(F) E(F)
Compression stockings and leg elevation reduce peripheral blood supply in patients with arterial insufficiency and they are therefore relatively contra-indicated. Surgical debridement may be required to excise necrotic and infected tissue. Femoro-distal bypass using autogenous vein improves peripheral arterial supply and helps ischaemic ulcer healing. Ligation of the sapheno femoral junction is used to treat varicose veins.

A17: A(T) B(F) C(T) D(F) E(T)

Epistaxis arises from the nasal septal vessels in most cases. It is associated with hypertension, atrophic rhinitis, tumours and bleeding disorders. If cocaine spray and cautery fail, then anterior pack of ribbon gauze soaked in paraffin is inserted. Foley catheter is used for posterior nasal bleeding where a 30 ml balloon lies in the posterior nasal space. Occasionally, anterior ligation is needed, e.g. maxillary artery, anterior ethmoidal artery and external carotid artery.

A18: A(F) B(T) C(T) D(T) E(F)

Extravasation of the sclerosing agent may cause skin damage and ulceration. Patients should be warned about the possibility of brown pigmentation of the skin. Sclerotherapy is indicated for residual or recurrent varicosities after varicose vein surgery. Sudeck's atrophy is a recognised complication of trauma.

A19: A(F) B(T) C(F) D(F) E(T)

BPH mainly affects the inner transitional zone. The outer peripheral zone is usually compressed and feels smooth to digital rectal examination. Any palpable nodule or irregularity should raise the possibility of malignancy. BPH seems to be an androgen-driven disease. Castration prior to puberty seems to prevent the disease. Alpha-blockers cause relaxation of smooth muscles and improve symptoms, whereas anticholinergic drugs could worsen symptoms and precipitate acute urinary retention.

A20: A(T) B(F) C(T) D(F) E(F)

Cystic hygromas are benign tumours of the lymphatics. The neck is the commonest location where these tumours could cause respiratory distress. Cystic hygromas may also occur in the axilla, groin and mediastinum. As they are benign tumours, important structures should not be sacrificed in order to achieve a complete clearance.

A21: A(F) B(T) C(T) D(T) E(T)

Interstitial cystitis is a disease of middle-aged women characterised by fibrosis of the bladder wall. Ureteric obstruction may be due to a stone fragment or a blood clot. Any clotting disorder should be corrected prior to PCNL. Since the advent of ESWL, the use of PCNL has decreased. 90% of renal calculi requiring intervention are now treated with ESWL.

A22: A(T) B(T) C(F) D(F) E(T)

Operations for lymphoedema can be classified into reducing or bypass operations. In reducing operations, the lymphoedematous subcutaneous tissue and skin are excised. In bypass operations, the sites of localised lymphatic obstruction are bypassed. Examples of reducing operations include Charles' and Homans' operations. Kinmonth's mesenteric bridge operation is an example of bypass procedures.

A23: A(T) B(F) C(T) D(T) E(F)

65% of thyroglossal cysts present before the age of 30 years. They usually present as midline swellings that move with swallowing. Laterally placed cysts are rare. The cysts may become infected and cause chronic discharge. Infected cysts are treated by needle aspiration and antimicrobials. The presence of lymphoid tissue in the wall makes such lesions susceptible to infection.

A24: A(F) B(T) C(F) D(T) E(F)

The patient is usually placed supine with 30° of head-down tilt to allow emptying of the veins. The operation is not recommended if the LSV is a collateral for obstructed deep veins, otherwise venous claudication may ensue. The LSV has approximately seven tributaries close to the SFJ. The femoral vein does not receive any tributaries except the LSV.

A25: A(T) B(F) C(F) D(F) E(T)

Intertrochanteric fractures cause shortening and external rotation of the leg. Adduction may occur due to unopposed action of the adductors. Hemiarthroplasty is more frequently performed for intracapsular fractures where the blood supply to the femoral head is more likely to be significantly compromised. In extracapsular fractures, the main blood supply is usually undisturbed and femoral head replacement is not necessary. In such cases DHS fixation is frequently performed.

A26: A(F) B(F) C(F) D(T) E(T) F(F)

Calcium carbonate and phosphate stones are the commonest salivary calculi. The submandibular gland with its tortuous duct is the commonest site of involvement. Surprisingly, the incidence of salivary calculi is increased by obsessional dental hygiene. It is thought that toothpaste fragments acts as a nidus for stone formation. Calculi near the end of a duct can be extracted transorally. Frequently a complete excision of the affected gland is required.

A27: A(F) B(T) C(T) D(F) E(F)

Primary hyperparathyroidism is caused by adenoma is most cases (90%). The clinical features are mainly due to the effects of hypercalcaemia. These features include renal calculi, constipation, bone cysts, pathological fractures, low serum phosphate, psychosis, etc. The presence of subperiosteal bone resorption of the phalanges is a diagnostic feature. Chronic renal failure may cause secondary and tertiary hyperparathyroidism.

A28: A(F) B(T) C(F) D(T) E(F)

Maldescended testis occurs in 2% of boys. The right-side is more commonly affected. Maldescended testes are usually hypoplastic. There is an increased incidence of malignancy, infection and trauma. Treatment is usually surgical with orchidopexy, such a treatment does not significantly reduce the malignancy risk. Other treatment modalities include human chorionic gonadotrophin (hCG) and LHRH analogues.

A29: A(F) B(F) C(F) D(F) E(F)

ESWL is currently used to treat more than 90% of renal stones. PCNL is still indicated in the presence of urinary obstruction not caused by the stone, for large volume stones and when the stone cannot be positioned within the focus of ESWL. Abdominal aortic aneurysms are a contraindication to ESWL.

A30: A(T) B(T) C(T) D(F) E(F)

Priapism refers to a sustained painful penile erection. Other causes include intercourse and idiopathic thrombosis of the prostatic veins. Conservative treatment modalities include noradrenaline, ganglion blockers and spinal anaesthesia. Surgical treatments entail the creation of a window between the glans/corpora spongiosum and corpora cavernosa. Impotence is a recognised complication of priapism.

A31: A(T) B(F) C(F) D(F) E(F)

Anaesthesia may be general, regional (Bier's block) or local into the fracture haematoma. The fracture is reduced by traction to overcome impaction, flexion to overcome dorsal angulation and ulnar deviation to overcome radial deviation. A plaster back slab is applied with wrist in slight flexion and the hand in ulnar deviation. The plaster is completed 6 days later, if the follow up x-ray shows a good position, in order to allow time for early oedema to resolve.

A32: A(F) B(T) C(T) D(F) E(T)
Colles' fracture is relatively common in post-menopausal women who have an increased incidence of osteoporosis. The fracture is reduced by traction (to overcome impaction) flexion (to overcome dorsal angulation) and ulnar deviation (to overcome radial deviation).

A33: A(F) B(F) C(F) D(T) E(T) F(T)
Smoking does not seem to increae the risk of breast cancer. Late menopause, early menarche and nulliparity increase the risk. Atypical epithelial hyperplasia increases the risk by five times.

A34: A(T) B(T) C(F) D(T) E(F)
Such a wound is bound to be infected. Initial management consists of debridement and thorough irrigation with normal saline. The wound is dressed regularly and closed 3–5 days later if it is clean.

A35: A(F) B(T) C(F) D(F) E(T)
Cervical spondylitis, cervical rib and neuritis of the median nerve should be considered as part of the differential diagnosis. Hypothyroidism but not thyrotoxicosis is a recognised cause. Other causes include diabetes mellitus, osteoarthritis, amyloidosis, drugs and Colles' fracture.

A36: A(T) B(T) C(T) D(F) E(F)
AVMs may lead to a high output of cardiac failure. The management of AVMs in growing children includes epiphyseal stapling to reduce limb irregularity. The management includes angiographic embolisation and surgical excision.

A37: A(F) B(F) C(T) D(F) E(T)
Pneumococcus is the commonest causative bacterium followed by *Haemophilus influenzae*. The latter is relatively common in children and treated with amoxycillin. Penicillin is used in adults. Tympanic membrane perforation is usually associated with relief of pain and fever. Myringotomy may be performed for painful bulging drums. In such cases hearing should be checked in six weeks.

A38: A(T) B(F) C(T) D(T) E(F)
Antibiotics do not seem to prevent rheumatic fever which is currently rare in Western countries. Quinsy refers to a peritonsillar abscess complicating acute tonsillitis. Retropharyngeal abscess is a rare complication. It requires incision and drainage under GA. The

use of antibiotics is controversial. If used, penicillin is the drug of choice as amoxycillin causes a rash if there is pharyngitis due to Epstein-Barr virus.

A39: A(F) B(T) C(T) D(T) E(F)
Simple cheek swelling may be due to a maxillary antral carcinoma or tooth root infection. Other clinical features include fever and cheek tenderness. Management consists of decongestants (ephedrine nasal drops), antibiotics (e.g. doxycycline) and analgesia.

A40: A(F) B(T) C(T) D(F) E(T)
Conjunctivitis is usually bilateral. The causes may be bacterial (purulent discharge), viral (adenoviruses) or allergic. Tetracycline (oral and topical) is the drug of choice in chlamydial infection.

A41: A(T) B(T) C(F) D(T) E(F)
Bilateral recurrent nerve injury (< 1%) may cause cyanosis and stridor but these signs may be due to other causes, e.g. cervical haematoma due to post-operative haemorrhage. Inadvertent injury or excision of the parathyroid glands may lead to hypocalcaemia and tetany. The vocal cords become adducted if the recurrent laryngeal nerve is injured. Bilateral injury causes stridor and cyanosis and is managed with endotracheal re-intubation or tracheostomy.

A42: A(F) B(F) C(T) D(F) E(T)
Thyroxine is mainly absorbed in the distal small bowel. The bioavailability of oral therapy is approximately 75% and 25% of the hormone is excreted in faeces. Its half-time is 6–7 days compared with 1–2 days for T3. T3 is less tightly bound to plasma proteins and has a quicker onset of action. Injectable preparations are available in some countries. The i.v. form is preferable as the hormone binds to muscle tissue.

A43: A(T) B(T) C(T) D(F) E(F)
The management of thyroid crisis includes intravenous fluids, cooling blankets, chlorpromazine, antidysarrhythmics, propylthiouracil (200 mg orally six-hourly), iodine (one hour following the first dose of propylthiouracil), lithium carbonate (in the presence of iodine sensitivity), propranolol (caution in patients with COAD or ischaemic heart disease), guanethidine, dexamethasone and plasmapheresis in severe unresponsive cases.

A44: A(F) B(T) C(F) D(F) E(T)
Superficial parotidectomy with an adequate margin of normal tissue is the treatment of choice. Enucleation with or without radiotherapy is associated with an unacceptable local recurrence rate. The role of pre-operative FNAC is controversial.

A45: A(T) B(F) C(F) D(F) E(F)
Wilms' tumour usually presents with weight loss and abdominal mass. Abdominal pain is often present but haematuria is a late presentation. Bilaterality indicates Stage V. The tumour is usually treated with a 5-day course of actinomycin D given pre-operatively, surgical resection and a post-operative course of vincristine. Radiotherapy is indicated in stages III, IV and V. One of the genes causing Wilms' tumour is located on 11p13.

A46: A(T) B(F) C(T) D(T) E(F)
The superficial inguinal region is the commonest site for an undescended testis. Other ectopic sites include perineal, femoral, penile and pelvic. Ectopy should be distinguished from crypto-orchidism in which the testis is arrested at some point in its normal descent.

A47: A(F) B(T) C(T) D(T) E(F)
The initial management of bleeding oesophageal varices includes resuscitation and insertion of a Sengstaken–Blackmoore tube which has four channels and two balloons. Other treatment modalities include portocaval shunting and oesophageal shunting.

A48: A(F) B(T) C(F) D(T) E(T)
Paraoesophageal hiatus hernias account for 10% of all hiatus hernias. The condition is rare before the fourth decade and is less likely to cause GORD than the sliding type. It may present as an emergency. Surgery is indicated once the condition is diagnosed.

A49: A(T) B(F) C(T) D(F) E(T) F(F)
Colonic pseudo-obstruction is a recognised complication of major surgery, opioids and major illness. The condition is usually associated with pain, particularly in the later stages. Treatment is initially conservative with fluid replacement, NG tube, nil by mouth and removal of precipitating cause if possible. Colonoscopic deflation is a recognised treatment modality. Caecostomy may be performed endoscopically, laparoscopically or through an open approach.

A50:   A(T)   B(F)   C(F)   D(T)   E(T)

Hot laparoscopic cholecystectomy can be performed in the first 72 hours. Acalculus cholecystitis may complicate trauma, sepsis and burns. The HIDA scan shows non-functioning gallbladder in acute cholecystitis.

A51:   A(F)   B(F)   C(F)   D(F)   E(T)

USS is helpful in confirming the diagnosis of acute pancreatitis, detecting gallstones and complications such as pseudocysts. Severity can be assessed by CT scanning which may show pancreatic necrosis indicating a severe attack. ERCP may play a therapeutic role in gallstone related pancreatitis. Octeotride (a somatostatin analogue) has not been convincingly shown to reduce mortality.

A52:   A(F)   B(T)   C(T)   D(T)   E(F)

Sigmoid volvulus occurs in a counter-clockwise direction. Young patients should be considered for a definitive treatment in the form of sigmoid colectomy once the first episode has resolved with non-operative treatment and the colon is prepared. Frail elderly patients may be treated with repeated sigmoidoscopic deflation. The recurrence rate with non-operative treatment is 50%. Hartman's procedure is indicated for gangrene and perforation.

A53:   A(F)   B(F)   C(T)   D(T)   E(T)

Gastrograffin swallow is the investigation of choice. Perforations measuring < 1 cm in size can be managed conservatively with antimicrobials, TPN and nil by mouth. Surgical repair is resorted to if the patient's condition deteriorates with conservative management. Surgical repair is also recommended for perforators exceeding 1 cm in size.

A54:   A(T)   B(F)   C(T)   D(T)   E(F)

Colonic perforation may complicate toxic megacolon. The incidence of colorectal carcinoma increases with duration of disease. The risk is approximately 17% at 20 years. Other complications include gastrointestinal haemorrhage, anal fissure and connective tissue disorder such as arthritis, uveitis and ascending sclerosing cholangitis. The latter can be treated with ursodeoxycholic acid.

A55:   A(T)   B(F)   C(F)   D(T)   E(T)

The FAP gene is located on the long arm of chromosome 5. Carcinoma complicates the condition in almost all cases by the age of 40 years. Prophylactic total colectomy prevents colorectal cancer.

A56: A(F) B(F) C(F) D(T) E(F)

K-ras oncogene is over-expressed in 80% of pancreatic tumours. Obstructive jaundice is not associated with a palpable gallbladder is more typical of gallstones. Operable tumours are treated by Whipple's operation. Radiotherapy and chemotherapy are not very effective treatment modalities. Palliative procedures include endoscopic stenting and surgical bypass. USS is not accurate in staging. CT scanning is more accurate. Other staging investigations include angiography, MRI, laparoscopy and intra-operative USS. Serum Ca19-9 is a tumour marker.

A57: A(F) B(T) C(T) D(T) E(F)

Injection sclerotherapy with 5% phenol is the treatment of choice for first degree haemorrhoids. Complications include haematuria, prostatitis and mucosal ulceration. Haemorrhoidectomy is the treatment of choice for third-degree haemorrhoids. The complications include pain and stenosis, haemorrhage and incontinence. Anal dilatation is associated with a high incidence of incontinence and should be avoided where possible.

A58: A(F) B(T) C(F) D(T) E(T)

Mixed gallstones containing cholesterol, bilirubin and calcium are the commonest variety. The incidence is increased in patients with inflammatory bowel disease. Symptomatic gallbladder calculi are treated by laparoscopic cholecystectomy in most cases. Non-invasive methods include oral chenodeoxycholic acid therapy and ESWL in selected cases.

A59: A(F) B(F) C(F) D(T) E(T)

Pancreatic pseudocysts consist of inflammatory products from neighbouring organs. The cyst takes 3–6 weeks to mature. The clinical features include a persistent rise in serum amylase, mild leukocytosis, low grade fever and abdominal ache. Small pseudocysts resolve spontaneously. Symptomatic and persistent pseudocysts can be treated by internal drainage (to stomach or jejunum) or percutaneous drainage under imaging-guidance. Complications of pseudocysts include peritonitis due to rupture and infection with abscess formation.

A60: A(F) B(T) C(T) D(T) E(F)

Dissolution therapy with chenodeoxycholic or ursodeoxycholic acid is indicated in infirm, elderly patients with symptomatic gallstones. The gallbladder should be functional and stones uncalcified. The recurrence rate is high. ESWL does not deal with the diseased gallbladder, therefore stones tend to recur after cessation of therapy. Internal drainage procedures are not advisable in the presence of sepsis.

A61: E
The most appropriate treatment in this patient is to drain the kidney through a percutaneous nephrostomy and administer antimicrobials.

A62: B
ESWL is now used to treat 90% of calculi which do not pass spontaneously.

A63: C
Cystine calculi dissolve in alkaline media. Other conservative measures include penicillamine and methionine administration.

A64: F
Calculi up to 5 mm in diameter usually pass out spontaneously. NSAIDs provide effective analgesia.

A65: D

A66: A
Cardiac pacemakers and abdominal aortic aneurysms are contraindications to ESWL.

A67: A
The tumour stage is T3N2a. Partial laryngectomy is inadequate, therefore total laryngectomy combined with neck dissection is the surgical treatment of choice. Radiotherapy may be given postoperatively. Chemotherapy is indicated for inoperable disease.

A68: B
Radiotherapy is as effective as surgery in the treatment of T1 tumours. However, the resulting voice quality is better than after surgery.

A69: F
Close monitoring is required.

A70: D
Vertical laryngectomy is more appropriate due to the increased risk of cartilage involvement.

A71: E

Nodal metastases are found in 55% of supraglottic tumours. Therefore, radical neck dissection, radiotherapy, or both is often required for large supraglottic tumours.

A72: D

Anti-thyroid drugs such as carbimazole are the treatment of choice in pregnant women. Such drugs can cross the placenta causing foetal goitre. Radioactive iodine is contraindicated.

A73: D

Patients under 18 years of age are best treated with anti-thyroid drugs initially. Radioactive iodine is contraindicated. Surgery is resorted to if medical treatment fails.

A74: B

Medical treatment has failed in this patient. Therefore, subtotal thyroid is the preferred treatment. Radioactive iodine is associated with a high incidence of hypothyroidism (up to 75%) and is preferable in women of child-bearing age.

A75: B

This patient seems to have Plummer's disease where the abnormality lies within the thyroid gland itself.

A76: F

The gland will usually regress in size unless there is considerable fibrosis. Surgery is indicated when a dominant mass is not suppressed by thyroxine therapy.

A77: A

The clinical features of weight loss, pain radiating to the back, obstructive jaundice, Troisier's sign and palpable gallbladder (Courvoisier's law) favour the diagnosis of pancreatic carcinoma. CT-guided biopsy and ERCP will help to establish the diagnosis.

A78: F

The recent history of laparoscopic cholecystectomy, the dilated CBD, the obstructive jaundice and the absence of sepsis make the diagnosis of retained CBD stone most likely. ERCP combined with sphincterotomy is indicated in this patient.

A79: D

This patient is medically unfit for major surgery or chemotherapy.

Radiotherapy is not effective in the treatment of hepatoma. Tamoxifen has been shown to prolong survival.

A80: A
This small hepatoma is suitable for surgical excision. Orthoptic liver transplantation is also a recognised treatment for a localised uninodular hepatoma in fit subjects.

A81: A
Hepatectomy for colorectal metastases can prolong survival. The 5-year survival rate is 25%.

A82: D

A83: E

A84: G
Gilbert's syndrome may present shortly after birth or several years later associated with intercurrent illness as in this case. Hyperbilirubinaemia is usually unconjugated and liver biopsy is normal. Serum bilirubin usually rises with fasting or intravenous nicotinamide administration.

A85: D
This patient seems to have ulcerative colitis and sclerosing cholangitis.

A86: I
The recent cholecystectomy and obstructive picture of jaundice make CBD stones the most likely diagnosis.

A87: C
The backache, the patient's age, the palpable gallbladder and acanthosis nigricans and superficial thrombophlebitis (migratory) suggest pancreatic carcinoma.

A88: A

System Modules Paper B

Questions

Q1   Recognised complications of chronic pancreatitis include:

A. Duodenal obstruction
B. Haemorrhage
C. Ascites
D. Pyoderma gangrenosum
E. Pseudocyst

Q2   Ischaemic colitis:

A. Is associated with collagen diseases
B. Presents early with abdominal distension
C. Commonly produces intramural gas which can be seen on plain AXR
D. Produces characteristic thumb printing on barium enema
E. Is usually treated by resection of affected bowel and primary anastomosis

Q3   Splenic rupture:

A. Is more common in patients with infectious mononucleosis
B. May be delayed for up to two weeks following blunt abdominal trauma
C. Should be suspected in patients with a raised hemidiaphragm
D. May displace the gastric air bubble on plain AXR
E. Produces a negative Kehr's sign

Q4   Anal fissure:

A. Is usually in the posterior midline in men
B. Is the commonest anal lesion in Crohn's disease
C. May be caused by *M. tuberculosis*
D. May be treated by topical GTN
E. May be treated by external sphincterotomy

Q5   Hereditary non-polyposis colonic cancer (HNPCC):

A. Accounts for 25% of colorectal cancers
B. Has an autosomal dominant inheritance
C. Usually presents in the 30–35 year age group
D. Produces tumours which are predominantly left-sided
E. Is associated with ovarian carcinoma

Q6   Pleomorphic adenoma of the parotid gland:

A. Is the commonest parotid tumour
B. Has a true capsule
C. Is a recognised cause of facial nerve palsy
D. Is effectively treated with radiotherapy
E. Does not recur after surgical excision

Q7   The long-term complications of renal transplantation include:

A. Hyperlipidaemia
B. Cerebrovascular disease
C. Hypoparathyroidism
D. Avascular necrosis of the femoral head
E. Cataracts

Q8   Anuria within 48 hours of renal transplantation is likely to be caused by:

A. Corticosteroids
B. Ureteric obstruction
C. Renal artery thrombosis
D. Acute tubular necrosis
E. Accelerated acute rejection

Q9   In the treatment of rectal cancer:

A. Excision of the mesorectum is not recommended
B. Pre-operative radiotherapy is contraindicated
C. 5-Fluorouracil is the chemotherapeutic agent of choice
D. A palliative defunctioning colostomy is the treatment of choice in the presence of liver metastases
E. The use of circular stapling devices has reduced the number of abdominoperineal excisions of the rectum

Q10   Oesophageal cancer:

A. Incidence is decreasing
B. Can be efficiently diagnosed with endoscopic abrasive cytology
C. Arising in Barrett's oesophagus is usually squamous cell carcinoma
D. Is associated with an overall five-year survival of 10%
E. Can be accurately staged with endoluminal ultrasonography

Q11   Bile duct injury after laparoscopic cholecystectomy:

A. Has a lower incidence than that observed after open cholecystectomy
B. Occurs approximately once in every 50 cases
C. Usually results from mistaking the CBD for the cystic duct
D. Is a recognised cause of biliary cirrhosis
E. May present with malabsorption

Q12   Ductal carcinoma *in situ* 'DCIS' of the breast:

A. Usually presents as a palpable mass
B. Can be distinguished from invasive carcinoma on fine needle aspiration cytology (FNAC)
C. Accounts for 17% of screen detected breast cancers
D. Is curable by total mastectomy
E. Is associated with axillary node metastases in 5% of cases
F. Is radio-resistant

Q13   The clinical features of acute pancreatitis include:

A. Carpopedal spasm
B. Cullen's sign
C. Reversed three sign on plain films
D. Elevated serum lipase
E. Acanthosis nigricans

Q14   A complete rectal prolapse:

A. Involves all layers of the rectal wall
B. Is relatively common in infants
C. Is commoner in males
D. May be complicated by gangrene of the rectum
E. May be treated with Délorme's procedure

Q15   When predicting prognosis in acute pancreatitis, Ransom's criteria at admission include:

A. Serum amylase level
B. Serum lactate dehydrogenase concentration
C. Serum lipase level
D. Patient's sex
E. White cell count
F. Serum potassium concentration
G. Blood glucose concentration
H. Patient's age over 55 years

Q16   Recognised complications of laparoscopic cholecystectomy include:

A. Small bowel obstruction
B. Pneumothorax
C. Incisional hernia
D. Enterocutaneous fistula

Q17   The clinical features of respiratory alkalosis include:

A. Hyperkalaemia
B. Tetany
C. Elevated serum bicarbonate
D. Carpopedal spasm
E. Shifting of the haemoglobin dissociation curve to the right

Q18   Transrectal ultrasonography (TRUS):

A. Is superior to suprapubic ultrasonography in measuring prostatic volume
B. Can detect 95% of prostatic cancers in the peripheral zone
C. Usually demonstrates a hypoechoic mass in the peripheral zone in patients with BPH
D. Can provide useful information in patients with azoospermia
E. Has an accuracy of 65% in staging prostatic cancer

Q19   Gastric carcinoma:

A. Arises in the greater curve in most cases
B. Is multifocal in 50% of cases
C. Is associated with *Helicobacter pylori* infection
D. Is resectable in most cases
E. Has a better prognosis than gastric lymphoma

Q20   Intussusception:

A. Is most frequently colo–colic
B. Produces passage of blood stained mucus as a late manifestation
C. In adolescence is frequently due to a Meckel's diverticulum
D. Is reducible by hydrostatic barium enema in 70% cases when performed with 24 hours of onset of symptoms
E. Is commonly recurrent

Q21   Recognised causes of acute abdominal pain include:

A. Myocardial infarction
B. Porphyria
C. Diabetic ketoacidosis
D. Lower lobe pneumonia
E. Viral hepatitis
F. Lead poisoning

Q22   Goserelin:

A. Is as effective as orchidectomy in the treatment of symptomatic metastatic prostatic cancer
B. Causes initial stimulation of the luteinising hormone release by the pituitary
C. Is indicated for management of advanced breast cancer in premenopausal
D. Is available as an oral preparation
E. Is a contraindication to the administration of cyproterone acetate in patients with advanced prostatic cancer

Q23   Hydrocele:

A. In infancy usually undergoes spontaneous closure in the second year
B. May contain bowel
C. May lead to testicular atrophy
D. In infancy, is usually treated by Lord's operation
E. Is a recognised complication of seminoma

Q24   Gas embolus is a recognised complication of:

A. Blood transfusion
B. Deep sea diving
C. Varicose vein surgery
D. Criminal abortion
E. Laparoscopic surgery

Q25   Prostatic specific antigen (PSA):

A. May be raised in patients with benign prostatic hyperplasia
B. Is a less sensitive serum marker for prostatic cancer than prostatic acid phosphatase (PAP)
C. Serum level greater than 1 ng/ml after radical prostatectomy is a sign of active disease
D. Is useful in estimating the tumour burden in patients with untreated prostate cancer
E. Pre-operative serum levels are very helpful in predicting the pathological stage of prostatic cancer

Q26   In the treatment of prostatic carcinoma:

A. Radical prostatectomy is indicated for a tumour staged T4 N2 M1
B. Radiotherapy is an appropriate treatment modality for a T4N0M0 tumour
C. LHRH agonists are effective
D. Radical prostatectomy is appropriate for a T2a tumour
E. Testosterone is a recognised treatment modality

Q27   Benign prostatic hyperplasia (BPH):

A. Mainly occurs in the outer caudal zone of the prostate
B. Causes a downward displacement of the veumonatanum towards the external sphincter
C. Is invariably progressive disease
D. Is a recognised cause of vesicoureteric reflux
E. Commonly causes the serum prostatic specific antigen (PSA) to be elevated above 50 ng/ml

Q28   Fat embolus is a recognised complication of:

A. Myocardial infarction
B. Pulmonary infarction
C. Morbid obesity
D. Closed femoral fracture
E. Total parenteral nutrition (TPN)

Q29   Recognised indications for liver transplantation include:

A. Primary biliary cirrhosis
B. Wilson's disease
C. Budd-Chiari syndrome
D. Familial hypercholesterolaemia
E. Primary hepatocellular carcinoma

Q30   The following criteria should be fulfilled in order to diagnose brain stem death:

A. Absent spinal reflexes
B. Absent spontaneous respiration
C. Absent carotid pulse
D. No gag reflex in response to pharyngeal stimulation
E. The pupils are fixed and unresponsive to bright light

Q31   Recognised complications of renal transplantation include:

A. Renal artery stenosis
B. Ureteric obstruction
C. Hypertension
D. Urethral diverticulum
E. Perivesical lipomatosis

Q32   The clinical features of acute epidymitis include:

A. Worsening of pain by gently lifting the scrotum
B. Urethral discharge
C. Prehn's sign
D. Reduced signal on colour flow Doppler sonography
E. Hydrocele

Q33   In transurethral resection of the prostate (TURP):

A. The bladder is moderately distended prior to resection
B. The chips in the bladder are washed out by isotonic normal saline during the operation
C. The proximal resection should include the fibromuscular fibres of the vesicle neck
D. The transurethral catheter is usually removed 24–48 hours post-operatively
E. Prostates larger than 90 g are particularly suitable for resection

Q34   In whole pancreas transplantation:

A. The pancreas is usually placed in the lesser sac
B. The exocrine secretion may be drained into the urinary bladder
C. Simultaneous renal transplantation is usually performed
D. The one year survival rate is less than 75%
E. The one year insulin independent rate is 60–75%

Q35   Irrigation of the bladder during TURP may cause:

A. Hyperkalaemia
B. Hypercalcaemia
C. Haemodilution
D. Hyponatraemia
E. Haemolysis

Q36   Recognised treatment modalities for colonic pseudo-obstruction include:

A. Oxybutynin
B. Colonoscopic decompression
C. Endoscopic caecostomy
D. Octreotide
E. Hydralazine

Q37   Hypospadias:

A. Results from incomplete fusion of the urethral folds
B. Occurs in one in every 900 male children
C. Incidence is decreased by taking oestrogen during pregnancy
D. Is associated with infertility
E. Is a contraindication to circumcision

Q38   Inguinal herniae in children are:

A. More commonly seen in children born prematurely
B. Commoner in females
C. A recognised cause of testicular atrophy
D. Treated by excision of the indirect sac and reinforcement of the posterior wall of the inguinal canal
E. Repaired only if they persist after the age of two years

Q39   Torsion of the testicle:

A. May be initiated by trauma
B. Is often accompanied by pyuria
C. May be diagnosed by ^{99m}Tc-pertechneate scintillation scanning
D. May be diagnosed with colour flow Doppler
E. Lasting for nine hours, must be treated with orchidectomy

Q40 Pleomorphic salivary gland adenomas:

A. Is usually treated by superficial parotidectomy
B. Can be diagnosed with fine needle aspiration cytology
C. Has a true capsule
D. May recur after surgical excision
E. Is highly radiosensitive
F. Is associated with smoking

Q41 Recognised complications of otitis media include:

A. Parotitis
B. Meningitis
C. Petrositis
D. Brain abscess
E. Facial nerve palsy

Q42 Parotid pleomorphic adenoma:

A. Is usually found in the deep part of the gland
B. Is most commonly superficial to the VIIth cranial nerve
C. Usually presents with a VIIth cranial nerve palsy
D. Is associated with 35% recurrence rate when treated by simple enucleation
E. Commonly undergoes malignant transformation
F. Is bilateral in 10% of cases

Q43 Recognised complications of abdominal aortic aneurysm repair include:

A. Trash foot
B. Ischaemic colitis
C. False aneurysm
D. Upper gastrointestinal haemorrhage
E. Chylous ascites

Q44 The following are recognised complications of a closed renal injury:

A. Renal artery stenosis
B. Urinoma
C. Haemorrhage from the kidney seven days after injury
D. The Page kidney
E. Medullary sponge kidney

Q45   Lignocaine:

A. Blocks the sodium/potassium pump in cell membranes
B. Depolarises nerve cell membranes
C. Does not affect motor nerves
D. Is a recognised cause of convulsions
E. Action is reduced by tissue inflammation

Q46   Occlusive disease of the femoral artery:

A. Most commonly presents with calf claudication
B. May cause Leriche's syndrome
C. Usually occurs at the level of the adductor hiatus
D. Can be treated with percutaneous transluminal angioplasty (PTA) if the occlusion is complete
E. Symptoms improve with nifedipine

Q47   Aorto-iliac occlusive disease:

A. Is a recognised cause of impotence
B. May present with a gangrenous toe
C. Treatment with axillofemoral bypass has a greater patency rate than aortobifemoral bypass
D. Causing complete occlusion can be treated with percutaneous transluminal angioplasty (PTA)
E. If unilateral, can be treated with femoro-femoral crossover graft in the unfit patient

Q48   Consequences of lower limb reperfusion following acute ischaemia include:

A. Decrease in serum creatine phosphokinase (CPK) levels
B. Metabolic alkalosis
C. Myoglobinuria
D. Acute tubular necrosis
E. Rise in intracompartment pressure of the calf compartment
F. Hyperkalaemia

Q49   Dissecting aneurysms of the aorta:

A. Usually arise because of cystic medial necrosis
B. Start in the descending aorta in most cases
C. Have an increased incidence in Marfan's syndrome
D. May cause electromechanical dissociation of the electrocardiogram (ECG)
E. Are usually accompanied by ECG changes suggestive of myocardial infarction (MI)

Q50   Treatments for Raynaud's disease include:

A. β-Blockers
B. Nifedipine
C. Ergot
D. Cervical sympathectomy
E. Naftidrofuryl oxalate

Q51   The following are recognised causes of mycotic aneurysms:

A. *Mycobacterium tuberculosis*
B. *Staphylococcus aureus*
C. Marfan's syndrome
D. *Salmonella*
E. *Trichophyton rubrum*

Q52   Buerger's disease:

A. Has equal sex distribution
B. Characteristically involves the medium-sized arteries of the extremities
C. Is a panarteritis
D. Will stabilise if the patient stops smoking
E. Causes foot claudication

Q53   The indications for carotid endarterectomy in patients with carotid stenosis include:

A. A complete stroke
B. Stroke in evolution
C. 50% stenosis without symptoms
D. 75% stenosis with a recent transient ischaemic attack
E. Amaurosis fugax with 75% stenosis

Q54   The complications of below-knee amputation include:

A. Neuroma of the posterior tibial nerve
B. True aneurysm of the popliteal artery
C. Phantom pain
D. Knee joint contractures
E. Gas gangrene

Q55   The following bones are particularly vulnerable to avascular necrosis following fracture:

A. Talus
B. Head of femur
C. Condyle of mandible
D. Scaphoid
E. Third metacarpal bone

Q56   The complications of tibial fractures include:

A. Fat embolus
B. Tibial nerve damage
C. Delayed union
D. Compartment syndrome
E. Leg shortening

Q57   Recognised complications of radiotherapy for breast cancer include:

A. Hodgkin's lymphoma
B. Lymphoedema of the arm
C. Breast sarcoma
D. Rib necrosis
E. Anaemia
F. Telengiectasia
G. Phyllodes tumour
H. Hamartoma

Q58   Mid-shaft femoral fractures:

A. Usually cause the proximal fragment to become extended
B. Usually cause the proximal fragment to become adducted
C. Usually cause the distal fragment to become abducted
D. Rarely cause sciatic nerve damage
E. Commonly cause significant blood loss due to profunda femoris vessel damage

Q59 In hand infections:

A. *Staphylococcus alba* is the commonest cause
B. Flexor tendon rupture is a recognised complication
C. Paronychial abscess is effectively treated with flucloxacillin
D. Palmar space abscess should be surgically drained
E. Primary suturing should never be performed following surgical drainage of tendon sheath abscesses

Q60 Supracondylar fractures of the humerus:

A. Usually result from direct violence
B. Frequently damage the brachial artery
C. Are usually reduced by traction on the distal fragment, followed by flexion at the elbow
D. Usually occur in children
E. Often cause ulnar nerve injury

Theme 1: Breast Cancer

A. Modified radical mastectomy
B. Radiotherapy and tamoxifen
C. Chemotherapy, radiotherapy and tamoxifen
D. Radiotherapy and aromatase inhibitors
E. Chemotherapy and LHRH analogues
F. Radiotherapy only

For each of the patients listed below, select the most likely single treatment from the options listed above. Each option may be used once, more than once or not at all.

Q61 A 51-year old woman presents with a 2.7 cm mass in the upper outer quadrant of the left breast. FNAC confirms malignancy. Mammography shows no other abnormality. Clinical examination reveals no evidence of metastatic disease. The patient undergoes wide local excision combined with axillary dissection. Histology demonstrates a 3 cm invasive ductal carcinoma which is completely excised (the closest margin is 1 cm). Three out of 10 lymph nodes contain metastatic carcinoma. The tumour is ER negative.

Q62 A 53-year old woman undergoes screening mammography which reveals a cluster of microcalcification on the upper inner quadrant of the right breast. Clinical examination demonstrates no abnormality. Stereotactic core biopsy reveals DCIS. A wire localisation biopsy is performed and histology shows a comedo-type DCIS which is completely excised. The ER status is negative.

Theme 2: Endocrine Tumours

A. Parathyroid adenoma
B. MEN type I
C. MEN type II
D. Carcinoid syndrome
E. Phaeochromocytoma
F. Medullary thyroid cancer
G. Parathyroid hyperplasia

For each of the patients described below, select the most likely diagnosis from the options listed above. Each option may be used once, more than once or not at all.

Q63   A 40-year old man presents with hypertension, palpitations and sweating. 24-hour urinary VMA is elevated. The lesion causing the symptoms is localised using an MIBG scan

Q64   A 25-year old woman presents with hypercalcaemia and bilateral nipple discharge. The various investigations reveal raised serum levels of parathyroid hormone and prolactin

Q65   A 40-year old man presents with recurrent episodes of flushing, colicky abdominal pain and asthma. Urinary 5-hydroxy indoleacetic acid (5HIAA) is found to be elevated

Q66   A 45-year old woman presents with hypercalcaemia and a thyroid goitre. Investigations reveal elevated serum levels of parathyroid hormone and calcitonin. Past medical history includes a right adrenalectomy three years previously

Q67   A 61-year old woman presents with stiff joints, myopathy and constipation. Plain radiographs reveal a right renal calculus and evidence of osteitis fibrosa cystica

Theme 3: Lower Limb Ischaemia

A. Femoropopliteal bypass
B. Percutaneous balloon angioplasty
C. Femorodistal bypass

D. Below knee amputation

E. Tissue plasminogen activator infusion (intra-arterial)

F. Fasciotomy

For each of the presentations listed below, select the most likely single treatment from the options listed above. Each option may be used once, more than once or not at all.

Q68 A 65-year old man presents with intermittent claudication of the left calf. The claudication distance is 100 metres. Angiography demonstrates a 1.5 cm stenosis of the left superficial femoral artery

Q69 A 73-year old diabetic woman presents with critical ischaemia of the right lower leg. Angiography reveals extensive disease of the superficial femoral, popliteal and tibial arteries. Pulse-generated run-off assessment indicates a good run-off in the posterior tibial artery

Q70 A 72-year old man presents with a four hour history of acute ischaemia of the left leg. Clinical examination demonstrates signs of acute ischaemia with no evidence of gangrene. There is no neurological deficit. An urgent angiogram reveals a complete occlusion of the distal superficial femoral artery most likely due to thrombosis

Q71 A 57-year old smoker presents with intermittent claudication of the right calf. The claudication distance is 70 metres. Angiography reveals a 12 cm stenosis in the proximal superficial femoral artery

Q72 A 21-year old motorcyclist presents with multiple injuries following a road traffic accident. Clinical examination reveals a critically ischaemic right lower leg. The right dorsalis pulse is feeble. The right calf is tense and swollen. The intra-compartmental pressure is 55 mmHg. Angiography shows no discontinuity of the arterial tree

Theme 4: Thyroid Cancer

A. Total thyroid lobectomy

B. Total thyroidectomy and removal of the central group of lymph nodes

C. Ablative dose of radioactive iodine

D. Reassure and repeat fine needle aspiration (FNA) in 12 months

E. External beam radiation

For each of the patients described below, select the most likely treatment from the options listed above. Each option may be used once, more than once or not at all.

Q73 A 40-year old woman presents with a solitary nodule in the right thyroid lobe. FNA cytology suggests follicular adenoma

Q74 A 20-year old woman presents with a 4 cm solid mass in the left thyroid lobe. FNA cytology reveals papillary carcinoma

Q75 A 15-year old boy presents with a 1 cm solitary thyroid nodule and diarrhoea. FNA cytology is reported as malignant Serum calcitonin is elevated

Q76 A 30-year old woman presents with a 2 cm thyroid nodule. FNA cytology suggests a colloid nodule.

Q77 A 50-year old woman presents with a thyroid goitre. A core biopsy reveals evidence of lymphoma

Theme 5: Colorectal Cancer

A. 5-Fluorouracil and radiotherapy
B. Hartmann's procedure and liver biopsy
C. Defunctioning loop ileostomy
D. Subtotal colectomy and ileorectal anastomosis plus left hepatectomy
E. Left hemicolectomy, primary anastomosis and left hepatectomy
F. Radical radiotherapy

For each of the patients described below, select the most likely single treatment from the options listed above. Each option may be used once, more than once or not at all.

Q78 An 84-year old man presents with complete large bowel obstruction. Plain abdominal x-ray demonstrates a grossly dilated colon (diameter 8 cm). Gastrograffin enema confirms complete obstruction at the distal sigmoid colon most likely due to a tumour. Abdominal ultrasonography shows four lesions in the left lobe of the liver suggestive of metastases. The patient's dehydration is corrected

Q79 A 59-year old woman presents with colovaginal fistula three weeks after anterior resection of the rectum for Dukes A carcinoma. Digital rectal examination shows no faecal impaction. Abdominal ultrasonography shows two echo free lesions in the left lobe of the liver and no evidence of collection in the abdomen or pelvis

Theme 6: Vascular Disease

A. Aortofemoral bypass
B. Percutaneous transluminal angioplasty (PTA)
C. Axillo-femoral bypass
D. Femoral-femoral cross-over graft
E. Lumbar sympathectomy
F. Ileo-femoral bypass
G. Femoropopliteal bypass
H. Femoro-tibial bypass

For each of the clinical cases listed below, select the most appropriate treatment from the list of options above. Each option may be used once, more than once or not at all.

Q80 A 70-year-old man presents with thigh claudication. Angiography demonstrates atherosclerotic narrowing of the distal aorta and proximal common iliac arteries.

Q81 An 83-year-old woman (smoker), presents with left thigh and buttock claudication. Angiography reveals a smooth narrowing (1.5 cm in length) in the left common iliac artery.

Q82 A 75-year-old man presents with severe right calf claudication. Angiogram shows narrowing (10 cm long) of the distal superficial femoral and popliteal arteries (right). The right posterior tibial artery has a reasonable run-off.

Q83 A 78-year-old man with severe emphysema presents with severe claudication of the left thigh and calf. Angiography reveals severe atherosclerosis affecting the left common and external iliac arteries. His past medical history includes previous anterior excision of the rectum and postoperative radiotherapy.

Theme 7: Skeletal Pain

A. Osteosarcoma
B. Ewing's sarcoma
C. Tuberculosis
D. Metastases
E. Multiple myeloma
F. Primary hyperparathyroidism

For each of the following clinical histories, select the most likely diagnosis from the list above. Each option may be used once, more than once or not at all.

Q84 A 70-year-old man presents with backache. Plain radiographs demonstrate multiple sclerotic areas in the lumbosacral spine.

Q85 A 50-year-old woman presents with backache and anaemia. Skeletal survey shows multiple lytic lesions in the skull and spine. Urine contains Bence-Jones proteins.

Q86 A 15-year-old boy presents with a painful swelling around the left knee. A plain x-ray shows a lytic lesion with sunburst appearance.

Q87 A 60-year-old woman presents with backache. Plain radiographs reveal osteoporosis, bony cysts and subperiosteal bone resorption.

Q88 A 70-year-old man with a history of Paget's disease of bone presents with a painful swelling of femur.

Answers

A1: A(T) B(T) C(T) D(F) E(T)
Duodenal obstruction is a rare complication. It is treated by pancreatic resection or gastroenterostomy. Pancreatic ascites is also a rare complication which may require pancreatic resection or Roux loop cover of leak. Pseudocysts complicating chronic pancreatitis are less likely to resolve spontaneously especially if size > 6 cm. Cystojejunostomy, cystogastrostomy or cyst duodenostomy may be performed to drain a pseudocyst.

A2: A(T) B(F) C(F) D(T) E(F)
Ischaemic colitis is frequently seen in elderly patients, post AAA repair, septic shock, SLE. Abdomen is usually tender and only later followed by abdominal distension. The most common radiological abnormality is the paucity of gas shadows in the bowel. Anastomosis is best avoided as there is a high incidence of break-down.

A3: A(T) B(T) C(T) D(T) E(F)
The spleen is more likely to rupture when pathologically enlarged. 75% of ruptures occur within two weeks. Displacement of the transverse mesocolon or gastric air bubble is occasionally seen. Referred pain over the left shoulder in the head-down position (Kehr's sign).

A4: A(T) B(T) C(T) D(T) E(F)
90% of anal fissures in men are in the posterior midline. Topical GTN for six weeks has healed nearly 70% of acute anal fissures. Lateral sphincterotomy is a recognised treatment of anal fissure.

A5: A(F) B(T) C(F) D(F) E(T)
Familial cancer accounting for 0.5–5% of colorectal cancers. Develops at 40–45 years. Has a better prognosis than sporadic cancers. Tumours tend to be more proximal, mucinous and poorly differentiated. Three HNPCC syndromes: Lynch 1, 2 (endometrial, gastric and ovarian cancer) and Muir Torre syndrome.

A6:   A(T) B(F) C(T) D(F) E(F)
Pleomorphic adenoma also known as mixed tumour, contains
stromal and epithelial elements. It accounts for 60% of all parotid
tumours. It is slow growing, but may be quite large at the time of
presentation. Facial nerve palsy is a rare complication. The tumour
is frequently multicentral and has no true capsule. Therefore, it
may recur after surgery. The latter aims at complete excision of the
tumour including a margin of normal parotid tissue. Radiotherapy
has no substantial role in treatment.

A7:   A(T) B(T) C(F) D(T) E(T)
Hyperlipidaemia occurs in up to 78% of patients. Avascular necrosis
of the hip or knee occurs in up to 10% of patients long-term,
probably as a result of corticosteroid therapy. Other long-term
complications include hypertension, coronary heart disease, malignancy, especially cutaneous and Cushing's syndrome.

A8:   A(F) B(T) C(T) D(T) E(T)
Azathioprine toxicity usually causes myelosuppression. Ureteric
obstruction and renal artery thrombosis should be diagnosed early
in order to salvage the transplanted kidney. Acute tubular necrosis
usually resolves in 7–14 days. Accelerated acute rejection is treated
by high doses of prednisolone but with a poor success rate for both
immediate and long-term graft survival.

A9:   A(F) B(F) C(T) D(F) E(T)
Excision of the mesorectum improves locoregional control and
probably survival. However, morbidity and the need for a
defunctioning loop ileostomy are increased in total mesorectal
excision.
    A short course of pre-operative radiotherapy may downstage
tumour and improve prognosis. The best palliative treatment for
metastatic colorectal carcinoma is excision of the primary tumour.
Hepatic resection, when indicated, seems to prolong survival.

A10: A(F) B(T) C(F) D(T) E(T)
The incidence of oesophageal cancer has been rising more rapidly
over the past decades. Patients usually present with advanced
disease, hence the overall five year survival rate is 10%. This
figure rises to 50% for early stage node-negative disease. Barrett's
oesophagus may be complicated by adenocarcinoma. The risk of
this complication depends upon the degree of cytological dys-
plasia. Radiotherapy and chemotherapy (given pre- or post-

operatively) have had a limited effect on prognosis. Endoscopic surveillance of high-risk patients remains the best method of improving survival.

A11: A(F) B(F) C(T) D(T) E(T)

The incidence of bile duct injury following laparoscopic cholecystectomy has been shown to be higher than that observed after open cholecystectomy (0.6 versus 0.3%). It occurs approximately once in every 200 cases. This incidence is too low for an individual surgeon to develop the skill and experience required to treat this difficult complication. The clinical features of bile duct injury include abdominal pain, fever, biliary fistula, malabsorption, recurrent cholangitis and secondary biliary cirrhosis, USS and ERCP are the initial investigations of choice.

A12: A(F) B(F) C(T) D(T) E(F) F(F)

In DCIS, the proliferating epithelial cells are confined to the ductal system without breaching the basement membrane. FNAC cannot tell us whether the basement membrane has been breached by malignant cells. DCIS accounts for less than 5% of symptomatic breast cancers and for 15–20% of breast cancers detecting with screening mammography. Less than 1% of DCIS lesions are associated with regional metastases. Mastectomy for DCIS is associated with a cure rate exceeding 99%. Recent trials have shown that radiotherapy is an effective treatment modality.

A13: A(T) B(T) C(T) D(T) E(F)

Carpopedal spasm is a feature of hypocalcaemia which may complicate acute pancreatitis. Retroperitoneal haemorrhage may cause Grey-Turner and Cullen's signs. Plain x-rays may show calcification (chronic pancreatitis) reverse 3 sign of the proximal small bowel and cut-off sign of the colon. Acanthosis nigricans indicates a visceral malignancy.

A14: A(T) B(F) C(F) D(T) E(T)

Partial rectal prolapse may be seen in young children due to excessive straining at defecation. It is usually self-limiting. Complete rectal prolapse is relatively common in elderly women. Délorme's procedure has a relatively high recurrence rate (40%). It can be performed under spinal epidural and local anaesthesia. It is of lesser magnitude than transabdominal rectopexy, which is the standard treatment in fit patients. Laparoscopic rectopexy has been tried recently.

A15: A(F) B(T) C(F) D(F) E(T) F(F) G(T) H(T)

Serum amylase concentration does not correlate with severity of acute pancreatitis. Other important prognostic indicators at 48 hours after admission include 10% drop in haematocrit, serum calcium under 8 mg/dl, hypoxaemia below 60 mmHg, anion base deficit > 4 mEq/litre and an increase of 5 mg/dl in blood urea nitrogen.

A16: A(T) B(T) C(T) D(T)

Small bowel obstruction may be due to adhesions, strangulated portal site hernia or gallstone ileus. The latter is a rare complication and seems to result from spillage of gallstones into the intra-peritoneal cavity. Inadvertent diathermy burn may result in an enterocutaneous fistula.

A17: A(F) B(T) C(F) D(T) E(F)

Hypocalcaemia ensuing from respiratory alkalosis may lead to tetany and carpopedal spasm. This can be corrected by rebreathing in a bag. Hypokalaemia is a feature of alkalosis. The $Hb–O_2$ dissociation curve is shifted to the right in acidosis.

A18: A(T) B(F) C(F) D(T) E(T)

TRUS is superior to digital rectal examination in the diagnosis and staging of prostatic cancer. Most prostatic cancer appears as hypo-echoic masses in the peripheral zone. However, 30% of cancers are isoechoic and 2% are hyperechoic. This means that TRUS can detect approximately two-thirds of prostatic cancers greater than 5 mm in size. In BPH transrectal ultrasonography shows sym-metrical enlargement of the transitional zone. TRUS is also useful in the assessment of the subfertile male.

A19: A(F) B(F) C(T) D(F) E(F)

Gastric carcinoma is commoner in the pre-pyloric region, antrum and lesser curve. It is multifocal in 12% of cases. Most cases are advanced at presentation and therefore are inoperable. Gastric lymphoma has a much better prognosis than carcinoma.

A20: A(F) B(T) C(T) D(T) E(F)

Intussusception is most frequently ileo-colic. When there is a delay in diagnosis > 24 hours, only 25% are reducible by barium enema. Intussusception is rarely recurrent, and is very difficult to diagnose. In the presence of a competent ileocaecal valve the intussusception may not be reduced by barium.

A21: A(T) B(T) C(T) D(T) E(T) F(T)
These medical causes of acute abdominal pain should be borne in mind when assessing patients.

A22: A(T) B(T) C(T) D(F) E(F)
Cyproterone acetate is often given concurrently with LHRH agonists in order to counteract the initial rise in androgen release. In the first two-three weeks of treatment, Goserelin is administered subcutaneously 10.8 mg every 12 weeks. Adverse effects include gynaecomastia (3%), hot flushes (50%) and nausea (5%).

A23: A(F) B(T) C(T) D(F) E(T)
Hydroceles diagnosed during infancy usually undergo spontaneous closure in the first year. If it persists beyond the first year, spontaneous closure is unlikely. In children inguinal incisions are used and the patent processus vaginalis is ligated at the internal ring and the distal sac is excised. Lord's procedure is appropriate in adults. Very tense large hydroceles may compromise testicular circulation.

A24: A(T) B(T) C(T) D(T) E(T)

A25: A(T) B(F) C(T) D(T) E(F)
PSA is also useful in monitoring patients after radical prostatectomy, radiotherapy and hormonal manipulation. Serum levels greater than 0.5 ng/ml three weeks after radical prostatectomy indicates residual disease. BPH can also raise serum PSA levels (by 0.3 ng/ml/g of BPH compared with 3.5 ng/ml/g of prostatic cancer).

A26: A(F) B(T) C(T) D(T) E(F)
The current treatment for T1 and T2 tumours is radical prostatectomy or radiotherapy. The former has a five-year disease free survival of 93% for T1 tumours and 85% for T2 tumours. Radiotherapy has a five-year DFS rate of 83% for T1 tumours and 70% for T2 tumours. Oestrogens, anti-androgens and LHRH agonists are used in the treatment of disseminated cancer.

A27: A(F) B(T) C(F) D(T) E(F)
BPH usually involves the inner cranial zone and is characterised histologically by hyperplasia of the acini and/or fibromuscular stoma. The earliest changes occur in the periurethral glands around the verumonatunum. Serum PSA rises by 0.3 ng/ml/gram of BPH compared with 3.5 ng/ml/gram of prostatic cancer, therefore it is uncommon for serum PSA to exceed 50 ng/ml in patients with BPH.

A28: A(F)   B(F)   C(F)   D(T)   E(F)

A29: A(T)   B(T)   C(T)   D(T)   E(T)
Other indications include primary sclerosing cholangitis, auto-immune chronic active hepatitis, fulminant hepatitis and α_1-anti-trypsin deficiency.

A30: A(F)   B(T)   C(F)   D(T)   E(T)
Other criteria essential to diagnosing brain stem death includes absent corneal reflexes, absent oculocephalic reflexes, absent vestibulo-ocular reflexes, no motor responsiveness within the cranial nerves and absent cough reflexes. The examination should be performed by two doctors (not from the transplant team) on two separate occasions.

A31: A(T)   B(T)   C(T)   D(F)   E(F)
Other complications of renal transplantation include rejection (hyperacute accelerated acute, acute and chronic), infections, glomerulonephritis, hypertension, hyperlipidaemia, coronary heart disease, cerebrovascular disease, malignancy (5.6% incidence) vascular necrosis of the hip and knee, obesity, Cushing's syndrome and cataracts.

A32: A(F)   B(T)   C(T)   D(F)   E(T)
Prehn's sign refers to the fact that scrotal pain is relieved by gently lifting the scrotum onto the symphysis. In testicular torsion, the pain worsened with this manoeuvre. Colour Doppler flow studies usually reveal an increased signal due to hypervascularity or inflammation.

A33: A(T)   B(F)   C(F)   D(T)   E(F)
During TURP, the first step is urethral calibration to reduce the incidence of post-operative strictures due to the use of too large rectoscope sheaths. The bladder is then moderately distended to define the prostatovesical junction and push the bladder walls out of the way in order to reduce the incidence of bladder wall injury. The proximal resection should be carried out to the level of the circular fibres of the bladder neck. Deeper resection can lead to bladder neck contracture. Non-electrolytic solutions, such as 2% glycine, are used to wash out chips. The three-way Foley catheter is usually removed 24–48 hours post-operatively. Prostates smaller than 90 g are more suitable for TURP.

A34: A(F) B(T) C(T) D(F) E(T)

The whole pancreas is usually placed in the left or right iliac fossa and the exocrine component is drained into the urinary bladder. Urinary amylase can be used as a guide to the development of rejection. The one-year survival rate is 90%. Diabetic patients frequently develop diabetic nephropathy and renal failure, therefore combined kidney, pancreas transplantation is frequently performed. Islet cell transplantation is an alternative method avoiding the problems of graft thrombosis and exocrine duct management, but the success rate is currently very low.

A35: A(F) B(F) C(T) D(T) E(T)

A dilutional hyponatraemia and haemodilution occurs because of absorption of the irrigation fluid into venous sinuses. Calcium is not a constituent of bladder irrigation solutions.

A36: A(F) B(T) C(T) D(F) E(F)

The initial management of pseudo-obstruction is initially conservative with i.v. fluid replacement, NG tube and nil by mouth. If a cause is identified, it should be corrected if possible. If this management fails, then colonoscopic decompression and/or caecostomy are considered. Caecostomy can be performed endoscopically, laparoscopically or as an open procedure.

A37: A(T) B(F) C(F) D(T) E(T)

Hypospadias occurs in 1 in 300 male children. It is evidence of feminisation and its incidence is increased by taking oestrogen and progestins during pregnancy. There are several forms of hypospadias: (1) glandular, (2) coronal, (3) shaft, (4) periscrotal and (5) perineal. The glandular and coronal forms are the commonest. Hypospadiac neonates should not be circumcised because the preputial skin may be used in future reconstruction.

A38: A(T) B(F) C(T) D(F) E(F)

The incidence of paediatric inguinal hernias is approximately 1-2%. The incidence rises to 5% in premature neonates. Males are more commonly affected. Inguinal hernias in children may become incarcerated causing bowel obstruction. In such cases, manual reduction can be achieved in 75%. Surgical repair consists of excision of the hernial sac (herniotomy). Venous infarction of the testis is a recognised complication.

A39: A(T) B(F) C(T) D(T) E(F)

^{9m}Tc-scintillation scan and colour Doppler sonography are helpful in differentiating the condition from epidimo-orchitis. In the latter condition, there is an increase in vascularity. Although torsion lasting longer than four hours is likely to lead to testicular atrophy, many testes remain viable after nine hours.

A40: A(T) B(T) C(F) D(T) E(F) F(F)

Pleomorphic adenoma usually arises in the superficial part of the parotid gland. It has no true capsule, hence the local recurrence rate after surgical excision. Simple enucleation has a higher recurrence rate than superficial parotidectomy.

A41: A(F) B(T) C(T) D(T) E(T)

Other complications include perforation of tympanic membrane, labarynthitis, subdural and extradural abscesses and mastoiditis. The incidence of these complications has decreased since the introduction of antibiotics.

A42: A(F) B(T) C(F) D(T) E(F) F(F)

Simple enucleation is associated with 20–45% recurrence rate. Annual incidence is 1.4 per 100 000. 60% occur in the tail of the parotid with the majority lying superficial to the facial nerve.

A43: A(T) B(T) C(T) D(T) E(T)

Trash foot is common after aortic operations. It is characterised by mottling and discolouration of the feet due to microemboli. Clinical ischaemic colitis complicates 1.5% of cases as it is associated with 50% mortality. Aortoenteric fistula is usually accompanied by infection of the grafts. Chylous ascites is a rare complication but, if persistent, may respond to perito-venous shunt.

A44: A(T) B(T) C(T) D(T) E(F)

The renal artery stenosis may lead to systemic hypertension. Urinoma refers to a localised collection (pseudocyst) of urine that has escaped into the surrounding tissue. Secondary haemorrhage due to lysis of the clot holding the renal fragments together is a recognised complication. The Page kidney is an ischaemic kidney surrounded by an organised haematoma.

A45: A(T) B(F) C(F) D(T) E(T)

Lignocaine is a weak base and therefore its action is reduced by the presence of acid which shifts the drug towards the ionised form. The latter does not penetrate cell membranes easily.

A46: A(T) B(F) C(T) D(F) E(F)
Liariche's syndrome refers to buttock/thigh claudication and impotence due to aorto-iliac disease. PTA is particularly suitable for short incomplete vascular stenoses. Occlusions which are complete, long or located at bifurcations are not suitable for PTA. Nifedepine is a calcium channel blocker that reduces blood pressure and peripheral blood flow.

A47: A(T) B(T) C(F) D(F) E(T)
Aortoiliac occlusive disease may present with buttock/thigh claudication, impotence or distal emboli (e.g. gangrenous toes). Short incomplete stenoses of the iliac arteries may be treated by PTA. Aortobifemoral bypass has a superior patency rate than axillofemoral bypass. In the unfit patient with unilateral disease, femoral-femoral cross-over graft is a less major procedure and can be performed under local anaesthesia.

A48: A(F) B(F) C(T) D(T) E(T) F(T)
Hypoxia due to hypoperfusion leads to cellular damage and anaerobic metabolism. Intracellular components are released into the systemic circulation including CPK, potassium, myoglobin, hydrogen ions and lactate. Compartment syndrome is also a feature due to oedema (intracompartment pressure exceeds 30 mm Hg)

A49: A(T) B(F) C(T) D(T) E(F)
Dissecting aneurysms of the aorta are usually due to cystic accumulation of mucopolysaccharides in the medial layer of the artery. They usually start in the ascending aorta and may cause cardiac tamponade. The condition is part of the differential diagnosis of MI.

A50: A(F) B(T) C(F) D(T) E(T)
β-Blockers and ergot may trigger Raynaud's phenomenon. Nifedipine (a calcium channel antagonist), cervical sympathectomy and naftidrofuryl oxalate (Praxiline) can improve the condition by causing cutaneous vasodilatation.

A51: A(T) B(T) C(F) D(T) E(F)

A52: A(F) B(T) C(F) D(T) E(T)
Buerger's disease usually affects young men who smoke. The major histological features of the disease occur in the intima and the media, and the advantitia are usually spared.

A53: A(F) B(T) C(F) D(T) E(T)

A54: A(T) B(F) C(T) D(T) E(T)
The incidences of neuroma formation can be reduced by cleanly dividing the nerve and allowing it to retract. Gas gangrene tends to occur in patients with peripheral vascular disease and its incidence can be reduced by the use of appropriate prophylactic antibiotics.

A55: A(T) B(T) C(F) D(T) E(F)
The blood supply comes from distal to proximal in the talus, scaphoid and head of the femur, predisposing them to avascular necrosis

A56: A(T) B(T) C(T) D(T) E(T)

A57: A(T) B(T) C(T) D(T) E(T) F(T) G(F) H(F)
Cancers complicating radiotherapy tend to occur 15–30 years after therapy. The incidences of lymphodema are particularly high if radiotherapy is given to the axilla following axillary clearance

A58: A(F) B(F) C(F) D(T) E(T)
The proximal fragment of mid-shaft fractures of the femur are usually flexed (unopposed action of the hip flexors), abducted and externally rotated (the action of the gluteus muscles which are inserted into the greater trochanter). This distal fragment is usually adducted.

A59: A(F) B(T) C(F) D(T) E(F)
Hand infections are usually caused by Streptococci and *Staphylococcus aurea*. Infections along the synovial sheath of tendons may cause shortening and rupture. Paronychial and palmar abscesses require surgical drainage and antibiotics alone and are not sufficient to cure the condition.

A60: A(F) B(T) C(T) D(T) E(F)
Supracondylar fractures of the humerus are relatively common among children and usually result from a fall on the outstretched hand. The brachial artery and median nerve may be damaged by the fracture. Brachial artery injury can lead to forearm pain and ischaemic contractures.

A61: C
Adjuvant chemotherapy is now indicated in all 'fit' patients with lymph node involvement. All post-menopausal patients should be prescribed tamoxifen (for 5–10 years), however the response rate is

lower in ER negative patients. Post-operative radiotherapy improves loco regional control after conservation surgery.

A62: F
Radiotherapy has been shown to be effective in reducing the recurrence rate (50% of recurrences are invasive) of DCIS following adequate local excision. It is particularly indicated in high grade DCIS.

A63: E
Phaeochromocytoma is also known as the 10% tumour. 10% of the lesions are located outside the adrenal glands, 10% are malignant and 10% are multiple. Inheritance may be autosomal dominant.

A64: B
This patient seems to have hyperprolactinaemia and hyperparathyroidism. MEN type I includes parathyroid adenoma, pituitary adenoma and pancreatic cell tumour.

A65: D

A66: C
This patients seems to have medullary thyroid cancer ($\uparrow$ calcitonin) and hyperparathyroidism. The previous history of adrenalectomy suggests phaeochromocytoma. MEN type II is the most likely diagnosis.

A67: A
The radiological investigations suggest hyperparathyroidism. Parathyroid adenoma is the commonest cause accounting for 90% of cases. Parathyroid hyperplasia accounts for approximately 10% of cases.

A68: B
Percutaneous balloon angioplasty is particularly suitable for localised stenoses and short occlusions. Lesions in the larger proximal vessels are technically easier to treat with fewer complications and the best long-term results.

A69: C
Femoro-distal bypass, using an autogenous vein graft, is the treatment of choice in this patient. The absence of images of the posterior tibial, anterior tibial and common peroneal arteries on angiography films must not be accepted as evidence of their occlusion.

A70: E
Intra-arterial thrombolysis with TPA or streptokinase is the treatment of choice in this patient, in view of the short history (four hours), absence of neurological deficit and angiographic findings.

A71: A
Such a long stenosis is unsuitable for angioplasty. Femoropopliteal bypass, using an autogenous vein or synthetic graft, is the treatment of choice.

A72: F
This patient has the compartment syndrome. Urgent fasciotomy is indicated in order to save his right leg.

A73: A
It is extremely difficult to distinguish between follicular adenoma and carcinoma on the basis of FNAC alone. Therefore a thyroid lobectomy is indicated.

A74: B
For small tumours < 1 cm, total lobectomy is a valid alternative. Post-surgery treatment includes radioactive iodine and suppressive thyroxine.

A75: B
This boy seems to have medullary carcinoma (most likely inherited). Investigations to exclude phaeochromocytoma and hyperparathyroidism should be performed prior to surgery.

A76: D
If the second FNAC is benign, then patient can be safely discharged.

A77: E

A78: B
Surgical excision of the primary colorectal cancer remains the best form of palliation. The lack of bowel preparation, the gross dilatation of colon and advanced age, favour Hartmann's procedure. However, complete bowel obstruction is not a contraindication to primary anastomosis as it is possible to perform an on-table colonic lavage. The liver lesions should be biopsied for histological confirmation. Left hepatectomy should be considered in the future and age alone is no contraindication.

A79: C
The most likely cause of this patient's fistula is anastamotic leak in view of the timing (three weeks post-operatively) and the Dukes stage. The liver lesions seem to be cystic on ultrasonography. A defunctioning loop ileostomy may succeed in closing the fistula. Radiotherapy and chemotherapy are indicated for Dukes B and C in appropriate patients.

A80: A
Aortobifemoral bypass using a synthetic graft is the treatment of choice.

A81: B
PTA is the treatment of choice for a smooth and short stenosis. The patient is advised to stop smoking and take aspirin regularly (75 mg).

A82: H
Femoro-distal bypass using autogenous vein (*in situ* or reversed) is the treatment of choice. This stenosis is too long for PTA.

A83: D
The previous colectomy and radiotherapy raise the possibility of severe adhesions which would make surgery on the aorta and iliac arteries difficult. In view of the severe emphysema, minimal surg-. ical intervention is recommended. Femoro-femoral cross-over graft can be performed under local or regional anaesthesia.

A84: D
The most likely diagnosis is metastases from prostatic carcinoma. The male sex, the patient's age and the sclerotic lesions are suggestive of the diagnosis. Serum PSA measurement may lend further support to the diagnosis.

A85: E
The multiple lytic lesions, anaemia and Bence-Jones proteins in urine make multiple myeloma most likely.

A86: A
The patient's age, the site of pain and swelling and the x-ray appearance suggest osteosarcoma.

A87: F
The diagnosis can be confirmed by measuring serum calcium and parathyroid hormone and performing a Sestamibi scan.

A88: A
Paget's disease of bone is associated with increased risk of osteosarcoma.

NOTES

NOTES

NOTES

NOTES

NOTES

NOTES

NOTES

NOTES

NOTES